DIAGNOSIS

Rare Medical Cases

VOLUME 2

EVERETT MILES, M.D.

FREE REIGN

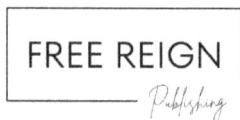

FREE REIGN
Publishing

CONTENTS

INTRODUCTION

Welcome to *Diagnosis: Rare Medical Cases*, a series that delves into the enigmatic and often perplexing world of rare medical conditions. I am Dr. Everett Miles, a practicing physician with over two decades of experience in internal medicine and diagnostics. Throughout my career, I have encountered a myriad of medical mysteries that have challenged the boundaries of my knowledge and expertise. This series aims to share these extraordinary cases with you, providing insight into the complexities and nuances of diagnosing and treating rare diseases.

Medicine is a field where every day brings new challenges, and sometimes those challenges come in the form of conditions so rare that they defy conventional medical wisdom. These cases often require not only a deep understanding of medical science but also an element of detective work, piecing together seemingly unrelated symptoms to arrive at a correct diagnosis. It is in these moments that the true art of medicine is revealed.

In each volume of this series, you will be taken on a journey through real-life cases that I have encountered in my practice. These stories are not only about the diseases themselves but also about the patients who lived through them. You will meet individuals who faced incredible odds, their courage and resilience shining through as they navigated the uncertain waters of their diagnoses. Their stories are a testament to the human spirit and the incredible advances in medical science that continue to evolve.

Each chapter will present a different case, detailing the patient's symptoms, the diagnostic process, and the eventual treatment. Along the way, I will provide insights into the medical thinking and decision-making processes that guided each case. You will gain a deeper understanding of how doctors approach complex cases and the importance of considering the rare and unusual when common diagnoses do not fit.

My hope is that this series will not only inform and educate but also inspire a greater appreciation for the intricacies of the human body and the remarkable field of medicine. Whether you are a medical professional, a student, or simply someone with a keen interest in medical science, I invite you to join me in exploring these fascinating and often bewildering medical mysteries.

Thank you for embarking on this journey with me. Together, we will uncover the stories behind some of the rarest and most intriguing medical cases ever encountered.

Dr. Everett Miles, MD

CARBAMOYL PHOSPHATE SYNTHETASE 1 DEFICIENCY

I had been a practicing pediatrician for over fifteen years when I encountered the patient with Carbamoyl Phosphate Synthetase 1 Deficiency (CPS1D), a rare and challenging urea cycle disorder. The patient was a three-day-old neonate, transferred to our hospital due to unexplained lethargy, vomiting, and rapid breathing.

Upon arrival, the patient was visibly unwell, displaying signs of severe metabolic distress. The initial workup revealed metabolic acidosis, hyperammonemia (ammonia level of 400 μmol/L), and respiratory alkalosis. Given the critical nature of hyperammonemia, our immediate goal was to reduce ammonia levels and stabilize the patient.

We commenced intravenous fluids with glucose to provide energy and reduce catabolism. However, the persistently high ammonia levels prompted further investigation. A thorough metabolic workup, including plasma amino acids, urine organic acids, and orotic acid, was ordered. Plasma amino acids showed markedly elevated glutamine levels, and the urine orotic acid was low, suggesting a proximal urea cycle defect.

Given the clinical presentation and laboratory findings, we suspected a urea cycle disorder. Genetic testing was initiated to identify the specific enzyme deficiency. Meanwhile, ammonia scavenging medications, such as sodium benzoate and sodium phenylacetate, were administered to help reduce ammonia levels. Additionally, we placed the patient on a protein-restricted diet and initiated parenteral nutrition to prevent further catabolism.

The genetic test results confirmed our suspicions: the patient had a mutation in the CPS1 gene, indicating Carbamoyl Phosphate Synthetase 1 Deficiency. CPS1 is the first enzyme of the urea cycle, responsible for converting ammonia into carbamoyl phosphate, a critical step in the detoxification of ammonia. Without functional CPS1, ammonia accumulates to toxic levels in the blood, leading to severe neurological damage and potentially fatal outcomes.

With the diagnosis confirmed, our treatment strategy focused on long-term management and prevention of hyperammonemia episodes. The following key components were incorporated into the treatment plan:

- Protein-Restricted Diet: We formulated a diet with minimal protein to reduce ammonia production. The patient was given essential amino acids and specialized formula to ensure adequate nutrition without overwhelming the impaired urea cycle.
- Ammonia Scavenging Drugs: Long-term administration of sodium benzoate and sodium phenylbutyrate was prescribed to help eliminate excess ammonia by alternative pathways. These drugs conjugate with glycine and glutamine, respectively, to form compounds that can be excreted in the urine.
- Arginine Supplementation: Arginine, an essential amino acid in CPS1D, was supplemented to support the residual urea cycle activity and enhance ammonia clearance.
- 4. **Regular Monitoring:** Frequent monitoring of plasma ammonia levels, liver function tests, and nutritional status was crucial. We established a schedule for regular blood draws and clinical assessments to catch any early signs of metabolic imbalance.
- Emergency Protocols: Detailed emergency protocols were provided to the parents and local healthcare providers. These included instructions for immediate hospital admission and administration of intravenous glucose and

ammonia scavengers during metabolic decompensation episodes.

Despite our comprehensive management plan, the patient's early months were fraught with challenges. Frequent hospital admissions were necessary to manage hyperammonemia episodes, often triggered by minor infections or dietary deviations. Each episode required intensive care, including dialysis on two occasions to rapidly lower dangerously high ammonia levels.

During one particularly severe episode, the patient developed encephalopathy with seizures. This incident underscored the critical importance of maintaining strict metabolic control and highlighted the fragility of patients with CPSıD.

Over time, with meticulous adherence to the dietary and medical regimen, the frequency and severity of hyperammonemia episodes decreased. The parents became adept at managing the complex dietary requirements and administering medications. Regular follow-ups showed gradual improvement in the patient's growth and development, albeit with some developmental delays.

At one-year-old, the patient underwent a comprehensive neurological assessment. While there were signs of mild to moderate developmental delay, particularly in motor skills and language, there was no evidence of severe neurological damage. Early intervention services, including physical and occupational therapy, were initiated to support the patient's developmental progress.

The patient's condition remained stable through meticulous management. However, the risk of metabolic decompensation persisted. The parents were vigilant, ready to respond to any signs of illness or metabolic imbalance. We worked closely with a multidisciplinary team, including dietitians, metabolic specialists, and genetic counselors, to provide comprehensive care.

By the age of five, the patient had experienced only a few minor hyperammonemia episodes, all managed effectively at home with emergency protocols. The developmental delays persisted, but with ongoing therapy, the patient made steady progress.

❧ 2 ❧
VALINEMIA

As a seasoned pediatrician with over two decades of experience, I have encountered numerous rare genetic disorders. However, a particular case involving a patient with Valinemia stands out due to its complexity and the rigorous diagnostic and treatment process it necessitated. Valinemia, a rare autosomal recessive metabolic disorder, presents unique challenges that require a multidisciplinary approach to manage effectively. This case not only tested my clinical skills but also underscored the importance of early diagnosis and comprehensive care.

❧

THE PATIENT, A THREE-MONTH-OLD MALE INFANT, WAS brought to my clinic by his parents, who were visibly anxious. They reported that the baby had been experiencing feeding difficulties, frequent vomiting, and failure to thrive. Additionally, they noted an unusual, sweet odor in the urine, reminiscent of maple syrup. This symptom immediately raised concerns about an inborn error of metabolism, specifically those related to branched-chain amino acids. Given the severity of the symptoms and the potential for rapid deterioration, I admitted the patient to the hospital for an in-depth evaluation and immediate stabilization.

Upon admission, the patient appeared lethargic, had poor muscle tone (hypotonia), and exhibited signs of dehydration. His weight was significantly below the expected percentile for his age, indicating failure to thrive. A detailed physical examination revealed no other overt congenital anomalies. However, the distinct maple syrup odor in the urine strongly suggested a metabolic disorder. With these initial findings, I initiated a comprehensive series of laboratory tests to pinpoint the exact nature of the metabolic imbalance.

- Blood Gas Analysis: The blood gas analysis revealed metabolic acidosis with a pH of 7.28, a bicarbonate level of 16 mmol/L, and an anion gap of 20. These findings indicated an accumulation of organic acids in the blood, a hallmark of metabolic disorders involving branched-chain amino acids.

- Serum Amino Acid Profile: Quantitative amino acid analysis showed markedly elevated levels of valine, leucine, and isoleucine. The levels of valine were particularly high, far exceeding the normal reference range, confirming our suspicion of a disorder related to the metabolism of branched-chain amino acids.
- Urine Organic Acids: Urine analysis revealed high levels of valine and its metabolites, including alpha-ketoisovaleric acid. The presence of these metabolites was consistent with a diagnosis of Valinemia.
- Genetic Testing: To confirm the diagnosis, we performed DNA sequencing, which identified a mutation in the BCKDHB gene. This gene encodes a subunit of the branched-chain alpha-keto acid dehydrogenase complex, essential for the catabolism of branched-chain amino acids. The identified mutation confirmed the diagnosis of Valinemia.

The combination of clinical symptoms, biochemical findings, and genetic analysis led to a definitive diagnosis of Valinemia. This disorder is characterized by a deficiency in the enzyme complex responsible for breaking down the amino acid valine, resulting in its accumulation and the subsequent buildup of toxic metabolites.

Valinemia is caused by a defect in the branched-chain alpha-keto acid dehydrogenase complex, specifically the BCKDHB gene. This enzyme complex plays a crucial role in the catabolism of the branched-chain amino acids valine, leucine, and isoleucine. When this enzyme is deficient or non-functional, these amino acids and their corresponding keto acids accumulate in the blood and tissues. The toxic metabolites interfere with cellular functions, leading to metabolic acidosis, neurological damage, and potentially fatal outcomes if not managed promptly.

The initial management focused on stabilizing the patient and preventing further metabolic decompensation. The following steps were taken:

- Intravenous Fluids: The patient was administered intravenous fluids to correct dehydration and metabolic acidosis. The fluids included a mixture of glucose and electrolytes to provide an alternative energy source and reduce the body's reliance on amino acid catabolism, thereby decreasing the production of toxic metabolites.
- Electrolyte Management: Frequent monitoring and correction of electrolyte imbalances were crucial. Bicarbonate was administered to manage the metabolic acidosis and maintain a stable blood pH.

- Emergency Medications: Sodium benzoate was administered to enhance the excretion of ammonia and other toxic metabolites through the formation of hippurate, which is easily excreted by the kidneys.

The cornerstone of long-term management for Valinemia is dietary control to limit the intake of valine and other branched-chain amino acids. A specialized metabolic dietician was consulted, and a comprehensive feeding regimen was developed:

- Low-Protein Diet: The patient was placed on a low-protein formula designed for metabolic disorders, which restricted valine intake while ensuring adequate nutrition. The formula was carefully measured to provide the necessary calories and nutrients without exceeding the safe levels of valine and other branched-chain amino acids.
- Specialized Amino Acid Supplements: To meet the patient's nutritional needs without exacerbating the metabolic disorder, essential amino acids, excluding valine, leucine, and isoleucine, were supplemented. This approach ensured the patient's growth and development were not compromised.

- Monitoring and Adjustments: The dietary plan required regular adjustments based on the patient's growth, development, and metabolic status. Frequent blood tests were performed to monitor amino acid levels, and dietary modifications were made accordingly to maintain metabolic stability.

Pharmacological interventions aimed to enhance the removal of toxic metabolites and support metabolic stability:

- Sodium Benzoate: Continued administration of sodium benzoate facilitated the excretion of ammonia and other toxic metabolites. The dosage was carefully adjusted based on the patient's blood ammonia levels to avoid toxicity.
- Carnitine: Carnitine supplementation was provided to support energy production and the metabolism of fatty acids, which can be impaired in metabolic disorders. Carnitine also helps in the transport of fatty acids into mitochondria, where they are oxidized for energy.
- Multivitamins and Co-factors: A comprehensive multivitamin supplement was given to prevent deficiencies that could arise

from the restricted diet. This included B-vitamins and other essential co-factors required for various metabolic pathways.

Regular monitoring was crucial to assess the effectiveness of the treatment plan and to make necessary adjustments:

- Frequent Blood Tests: Regular blood tests were conducted to monitor amino acid levels, blood gases, and electrolytes. This allowed for early detection of metabolic imbalances and prompt intervention.
- Growth and Development Assessments: The patient's growth parameters, including weight, height, and head circumference, were closely monitored. Developmental milestones were assessed to ensure the patient was achieving age-appropriate skills.
- Neurological Assessments: Given the risk of neurological damage in Valinemia, regular neurological assessments were performed. These included evaluations of motor skills, cognitive development, and behavioral observations.

During the course of treatment, the patient experienced several complications that required prompt intervention:

- Metabolic Crises: The patient occasionally experienced episodes of metabolic decompensation, often triggered by infections or dietary indiscretions. These episodes presented with increased lethargy, vomiting, and metabolic acidosis. During these crises, the patient was admitted to the hospital for intensive management, which included intravenous fluids, glucose, and adjustments to the dietary plan. Emergency medications like sodium benzoate and bicarbonate were administered to stabilize the patient.
- Growth Delays: Despite careful dietary management, the patient exhibited growth delays. This was addressed by increasing calorie intake and ensuring the diet provided adequate nutrients to support growth. High-calorie supplements and specialized formulas were used to promote weight gain and overall growth.
- Nutritional Deficiencies: The restricted diet posed a risk of nutritional deficiencies. Regular blood tests were conducted to monitor levels of essential vitamins and minerals. Supplementation was adjusted based

on these results to prevent deficiencies and support optimal health.

After several months of rigorous management, the patient's condition stabilized. The parents were educated on the importance of adhering to the dietary restrictions and recognizing early signs of metabolic crises. They were provided with detailed instructions on how to manage the diet at home and what steps to take in case of an emergency. With consistent care and monitoring, the patient showed improvement in growth and developmental parameters, albeit with some ongoing challenges.

Valinemia, being a chronic condition, requires lifelong management. The prognosis largely depends on early diagnosis, strict adherence to dietary and pharmacological treatments, and regular monitoring. With proper management, many patients can lead relatively normal lives, although they remain at risk for metabolic crises and neurological complications. The patient's parents were made aware of the need for continuous follow-up and were connected with a support group for families dealing with metabolic disorders.

Through coordinated efforts involving dieticians, geneticists, and pediatricians, we were able to stabilize the patient and improve the quality of life.

DANON DISEASE

The patient first came to my clinic with complaints of progressive muscle weakness, fatigue, and heart palpitations. At the age of 16, such symptoms were unusual and concerning. During the initial physical examination, I noted that the patient had hypertrophic cardiomyopathy, characterized by a thickened heart muscle that obstructs blood flow. This finding necessitated further investigation, given the severity of the symptoms and the potential for a life-threatening condition.

After discussing the findings with the patient and their family, we proceeded with a series of diagnostic tests. The first step was to perform an echocardiogram to get a detailed view of the heart's structure and function. The echocardiogram confirmed significant hypertrophy of the left ventricle, with an ejection fraction slightly below normal. This confirmed the suspicion of hypertrophic cardiomyopathy.

Given the rarity of hypertrophic cardiomyopathy in such a young patient, I ordered a genetic panel to screen for mutations commonly associated with cardiomyopathies. While awaiting the results, we initiated treatment to manage the patient's symptoms and prevent complications. The patient was started on a beta-blocker, metoprolol, at a dose of 50 mg twice daily, to reduce the heart rate and myocardial oxygen demand. Additionally, I prescribed an ACE inhibitor, enalapril, 10 mg daily, to help manage blood pressure and reduce the workload on the heart.

Within two weeks, the genetic testing results arrived. They revealed a mutation in the LAMP2 gene, confirming a diagnosis of Danon disease. Danon disease is an X-linked lysosomal storage disorder characterized by the triad of cardiomyopathy, skeletal myopathy, and intellectual disability. This explained the patient's symptoms and provided a clear direction for further management.

The next step was to assess the extent of the patient's skeletal muscle involvement. A muscle biopsy was performed, which showed vacuolar myopathy with autophagic vacuoles and glycogen accumulation, consistent with Danon disease. The muscle weakness the patient experienced was a direct result of these pathological changes in the muscle tissue.

To manage the cardiac aspect of Danon disease, we referred the patient to a cardiologist specializing in inherited cardiomyopathies. The cardiologist recommended the continuation of the current medications and added spironolactone, 25 mg daily, to prevent heart failure progression by blocking aldosterone, a hormone that can contribute to heart muscle fibrosis.

Given the progressive nature of Danon disease, we also discussed the possibility of advanced therapies with the patient and their family. One such therapy was the consideration of a heart transplant. The cardiologist initiated the process of evaluating the patient for heart transplantation, including consultations with a transplant surgeon and a detailed evaluation of the patient's overall health status.

During this period, the patient began experiencing increased difficulty with physical activities, such as climbing stairs and even walking short distances. Physical therapy was initiated to help maintain muscle function and improve the patient's quality of life. The physical therapist designed a tailored exercise program focusing on low-impact aerobic exercises and muscle strengthening routines to address the muscle weakness.

In parallel, we explored experimental treatments and clinical trials for Danon disease. The patient enrolled in a clinical trial investigating the efficacy of gene therapy targeting the LAMP2 mutation. This involved regular visits to the research center for monitoring and administration of the investigational therapy.

Despite our efforts, the patient's cardiac function continued to deteriorate over the following months. The patient was hospitalized multiple times for heart failure exacerbations, requiring intravenous diuretics to manage fluid overload and improve breathing. During one of these hospitalizations, the patient developed ventricular tachycardia, a potentially fatal arrhythmia. An implantable cardioverter-defibrillator (ICD) was placed to prevent sudden cardiac death by detecting and correcting life-threatening arrhythmias.

The decline in the patient's cardiac function was paralleled by worsening skeletal muscle weakness. The patient struggled with daily activities and became increasingly reliant on assistive devices, such as a wheelchair, for mobility. Occupational therapy was incorporated into the patient's care plan to help adapt the home environment and provide tools to assist with daily tasks, aiming to preserve as much independence as possible.

Six months into the clinical trial, preliminary results showed some promise in slowing the progression of the disease, but the patient's condition remained critical. The patient's family faced difficult decisions regarding the continuation of aggressive treatments versus focusing on palliative care to ensure comfort in the remaining time.

As the patient's primary care physician, I facilitated

numerous discussions with the family about the prognosis and the realistic expectations of treatment outcomes. These conversations were heart-wrenching but necessary to align the medical interventions with the patient's wishes and quality of life goals. It became evident that the patient's heart function was unlikely to improve without a transplant, and even with a transplant, the long-term outlook was uncertain given the systemic nature of Danon disease.

Ultimately, the patient's heart function declined to the point where they were listed for a heart transplant. The wait for a suitable donor heart was agonizing, and the patient's condition required continuous inotropic support to maintain cardiac output. Despite being on the transplant list, the patient's overall health continued to worsen, with frequent hospital admissions for decompensated heart failure.

During this time, we also addressed the patient's nutritional needs. Danon disease can lead to gastrointestinal complications, including delayed gastric emptying and malabsorption. A dietitian was consulted to develop a high-calorie, nutrient-dense diet plan to counteract the patient's muscle wasting and weight loss. This plan included easily digestible foods and supplements to ensure adequate protein intake.

In addition to the physical challenges, the patient and their family faced significant emotional and psychological burdens. A psychologist specializing in chronic illness was brought in to provide counseling and support. These sessions focused on coping strategies, stress management, and addressing the anticipatory grief associated with the patient's declining health.

In the final months, the patient was transitioned to hospice care. The focus shifted to managing symptoms and providing emotional support to the patient and their family. Medications were adjusted to ensure comfort, and the patient received regular visits from a multidisciplinary hospice team, including nurses, social workers, and chaplains.

The hospice team worked closely with the family to manage the patient's symptoms at home. This included adjusting medications to alleviate pain, shortness of breath, and anxiety. The use of morphine and lorazepam was carefully titrated to ensure the patient's comfort without causing excessive sedation. The goal was to allow the patient to spend meaningful time with family and friends in a familiar environment.

Throughout the hospice care period, we maintained open communication with the family, providing regular updates on the patient's condition and addressing any concerns. The hospice team also provided education on what to expect in the final stages of life, helping the family prepare for the inevitable while ensuring that the patient's dignity and preferences were respected.

The patient passed away peacefully surrounded by family. Despite the aggressive interventions and participation in cutting-edge research, the progressive nature of Danon disease and the severe cardiac involvement ultimately led to the patient's demise.

Following the patient's death, a thorough review of the case was conducted. This included a detailed analysis of the clinical course, treatment interventions, and the patient's response to various therapies. The findings were presented at a multidisciplinary conference to share insights and discuss potential improvements in the management of Danon disease.

The genetic component of Danon disease also prompted a discussion with the patient's family about genetic counseling and testing. Since Danon disease is inherited in an X-linked manner, there was a risk of other family members being affected or being carriers of the mutation. Genetic counseling sessions were arranged to provide the family with information on inheritance patterns, testing options, and reproductive choices.

From a scientific perspective, this case highlighted the need for continued research into the underlying mechanisms of Danon disease and the development of targeted therapies. The involvement in the gene therapy trial, although ultimately not curative for the patient, provided valuable data that could inform future treatments and potentially offer hope for others with this devastating condition.

In summary, managing the patient's journey through Danon disease was a profound and challenging experience. It required a comprehensive approach that addressed the complex interplay of cardiac, skeletal muscle, and psychological aspects the disease. The collaborative efforts of a multidisciplinary team were crucial in providing holistic care and supporting the patient and their family through every stage of the illness.

✤ 4 ✤
URTICARIA, COLD

I first encountered the patient on a brisk January morning, their face flushed from the biting cold. They appeared anxious, scratching at their forearms and cheeks with fervor. The initial consultation began with the patient describing their symptoms: an intense itching sensation and raised, red welts that appeared after exposure to cold environments. The welts subsided gradually once they were back in warmer conditions.

Upon hearing these symptoms, I immediately suspected cold urticaria, a relatively rare type of physical urticaria triggered by exposure to cold air, water, or objects. To confirm my hypothesis, I conducted a thorough history and physical examination.

1. History:

- The patient reported a history of recurrent episodes of itching and hives upon exposure to cold weather, particularly in winter months.
- They described incidents where cold drinks caused swelling in their throat, leading to difficulty swallowing.
- There was no significant family history of similar symptoms, allergies, or atopy.
- The patient denied any recent infections, new medications, or travel history that might have introduced new allergens.

2. Physical Examination:

- Vital signs were within normal limits.
- Dermatological examination revealed erythematous, raised wheals on the forearms and cheeks. The distribution pattern was consistent with areas exposed to the cold.
- There were no signs of angioedema in the periorbital or perioral regions.

3. Diagnostic Testing:

- A cold stimulation test, which involves placing an ice cube on the forearm for 5 minutes, was performed. Within a few minutes of removing the ice, a distinct wheal developed at the site of contact, confirming cold urticaria.

- Blood tests, including a complete blood count (CBC), liver function tests (LFTs), renal function tests (RFTs), and thyroid function tests (TFTs), were ordered to rule out underlying systemic conditions. All results were within normal ranges.
- Immunoglobulin E (IgE) levels were slightly elevated, but not significantly.

With the diagnosis of cold urticaria confirmed, the next step was to develop a comprehensive treatment plan. Cold urticaria management primarily involves avoiding exposure to cold and symptomatic treatment.

1. Patient Education and Avoidance Strategies:

- I advised the patient to avoid sudden temperature changes and to keep their body warm, particularly when going outdoors in cold weather.
- They were instructed to avoid consuming cold foods and beverages, which could trigger oropharyngeal edema.
- The patient was informed about the importance of carrying an emergency kit containing antihistamines and an epinephrine

auto-injector, especially when exposure to cold could not be avoided.

2. Pharmacological Treatment:

- Antihistamines: The patient was prescribed a second-generation antihistamine, cetirizine, at a dose of 10 mg daily. Second-generation antihistamines are preferred due to their lower sedative effects compared to first-generation antihistamines.
- Montelukast: Considering the potential involvement of leukotrienes in cold urticaria, I added montelukast, a leukotriene receptor antagonist, at a dose of 10 mg daily.
- Epinephrine Auto-Injector: Given the risk of anaphylaxis, particularly with systemic exposure to cold (such as swimming in cold water), I prescribed an epinephrine auto-injector (0.3 mg). The patient was trained on its proper use and instructed to seek immediate medical attention if they ever needed to use it.

3. Follow-Up and Monitoring:

- A follow-up appointment was scheduled for one month later to assess the efficacy of the treatment and make any necessary adjustments.

- The patient was advised to maintain a symptom diary, recording instances of cold exposure, the severity of symptoms, and any use of medications.

At the one-month follow-up, the patient reported a significant reduction in the frequency and severity of their symptoms. They had adhered to the avoidance strategies, wearing appropriate clothing to protect against the cold and avoiding cold foods and drinks. The cetirizine and montelukast combination effectively managed their symptoms, with only occasional mild itching occurring despite strict avoidance.

However, the patient experienced one episode where they inadvertently came into contact with cold water while washing their hands, resulting in localized hives and mild swelling. They managed this episode with the emergency antihistamine in their kit, without the need for epinephrine.

Given the positive response to treatment, the patient was advised to continue the current regimen of cetirizine and montelukast. They were reminded of the importance of avoiding cold exposure and carrying their emergency kit at all times.

Cold urticaria is a chronic condition that can persist for several years, with some patients experiencing spontaneous remission. The mainstay of management is ongoing avoidance of triggers and symptomatic treatment. I provided the patient with the following long-term management plan:

1. Regular Follow-Up:

- Periodic follow-up visits were scheduled every 3 to 6 months to monitor symptoms and adjust treatment as necessary.

2. Continued Education:

- The patient was encouraged to stay informed about their condition and to seek medical advice promptly if they experienced any changes in symptoms or required frequent use of their emergency medications.

3. Potential Desensitization:

- For patients with severe or refractory cold urticaria, desensitization therapy through gradual and controlled exposure to cold can be considered. However, this approach requires careful supervision and is typically reserved for those who do not respond to standard treatments.

4. Evaluation for Underlying Conditions:

- Although the patient's initial workup did not reveal any underlying systemic conditions, I advised that they undergo periodic evaluations to ensure no new conditions develop that might contribute to their symptoms.

Over the course of several years, the patient continued to manage their cold urticaria effectively with the combination of avoidance strategies and pharmacotherapy. They remained vigilant about their condition, adhering to the recommendations provided. The patient's quality of life improved significantly, and they experienced fewer and less severe episodes of urticaria.

Through meticulous diagnosis, comprehensive patient education, and a tailored treatment plan, the patient was able to achieve and maintain good control over their cold urticaria. The patient did not experience any life-threatening episodes and was able to lead a relatively normal life with the appropriate precautions and medications.

❧ 5 ❧
ENTEROBIASIS

When the patient first entered my office, they appeared visibly distressed. It was a busy Tuesday afternoon in the clinic, and I could tell from their agitation that something was seriously bothering them. I asked them to sit down and to describe their symptoms in as much detail as possible.

The patient, a middle-aged adult, explained that they had been experiencing severe itching in the anal area for the past several nights. This itching was most intense at night and had been progressively worsening over the past week. They also mentioned noticing small, white, thread-like worms in their stool and around the anal area, which alarmed them greatly.

From the patient's description, I suspected Enterobiasis, a common parasitic infection caused by the pinworm, Enterobius vermicularis. Enterobiasis is particularly prevalent in children but can affect individuals of any age. The intense nocturnal itching is due to the female pinworms migrating to the perianal region to lay their eggs.

To confirm the diagnosis, I explained to the patient that we would need to perform a few diagnostic tests. I first conducted a visual examination of the perianal region, where I observed signs of inflammation and irritation consistent with pinworm infection. Next, I performed the "tape test." This simple diagnostic method involves applying a piece of transparent adhesive tape to the perianal area early in the morning before the patient has bathed or used the bathroom. The tape is then placed on a glass slide and examined under a microscope.

As expected, the tape test revealed the presence of pinworm eggs, confirming the diagnosis of Enterobiasis. The eggs are oval, slightly flattened on one side, and have a characteristic thick shell, making them easily identifiable under microscopic examination.

With the diagnosis confirmed, I moved on to discussing the treatment plan with the patient. Enterobiasis is usually treated with anthelmintic medications, which are effective in eradicating the infection. The two most commonly used medications are mebendazole and albendazole. Both medications are available in single-dose regimens, which are typically repeated after two weeks to ensure complete eradication of the infection and to kill any newly hatched worms.

I prescribed a single dose of 100 mg of mebendazole, with instructions to take the medication immediately and to repeat the dose in two weeks. Mebendazole works by inhibiting the microtubule synthesis of the worms, effectively disrupting their cellular structures and causing their death. This medication is generally well-tolerated, with minimal side effects, although some patients may experience mild gastrointestinal disturbances such as nausea or abdominal pain.

In addition to the medication, I provided the patient with comprehensive hygiene measures to prevent rein-fection and to reduce the risk of spreading the infection to others. These measures included:

- Personal Hygiene: Emphasizing the importance of thorough handwashing with soap and water, especially after using the toilet and before meals. The patient was advised to keep their fingernails short and to avoid scratching the perianal area to minimize the risk of spreading the eggs.
- Laundry and Bedding: I instructed the patient to wash all bedding, clothing, and towels in hot water and to dry them on high heat to kill any pinworm eggs. Bed linens and underwear

should be changed daily during the treatment period.

- Household Cleaning: I recommended daily vacuuming or mopping of the floors in the bedroom and bathroom to remove any eggs that may have been dispersed in the environment. Surfaces such as toilet seats, doorknobs, and countertops should be cleaned regularly with disinfectant.
- Family Members: Given the high likelihood of transmission within households, I advised that all family members be treated simultaneously, even if they were asymptomatic. This approach helps to prevent the cycle of reinfection that can occur in close living quarters.

I scheduled a follow-up appointment for the patient in four weeks to assess the effectiveness of the treatment and to ensure that the infection had been fully eradicated. During this period, I encouraged the patient to maintain diligent hygiene practices and to monitor for any recurrence of symptoms.

At the follow-up appointment, the patient reported significant improvement. The intense nocturnal itching had subsided within a few days of starting the treatment, and they had not observed any further presence of worms. I performed another tape test to confirm the absence of pinworm eggs, and the results were negative, indicating that the infection had been successfully treated.

However, I emphasized the importance of continued vigilance and hygiene measures to prevent future infections. Enterobiasis is highly contagious, and reinfection is common if preventive measures are not strictly followed. I advised the patient to maintain good personal hygiene, to continue regular cleaning of their living environment, and to be mindful of the potential for transmission in communal settings such as schools or daycares.

The patient's case of Enterobiasis was successfully diagnosed and treated with a combination of anthelmintic medication and stringent hygiene measures. The patient recovered fully without any complications, highlighting the effectiveness of a comprehensive approach to managing this common parasitic infection.

❧ 6 ❧
TAKOTSUBO CARDIOMYOPATHY

When the patient arrived at the emergency room, their symptoms were strikingly similar to those of a myocardial infarction. They were a middle-aged individual presenting with acute chest pain, dyspnea, and diaphoresis. The initial ECG revealed ST-segment elevation in the anterior leads, prompting an immediate response in our protocol for acute coronary syndrome (ACS).

Given the gravity of the situation, we proceeded with an emergent coronary angiography to evaluate the state of the coronary arteries. Remarkably, the angiogram revealed no significant obstructive coronary artery disease. This finding was incongruent with the patient's clinical presentation and the ECG changes, necessitating further investigation.

Considering the differential diagnosis, we contemplated Takotsubo cardiomyopathy, also known as stress-induced cardiomyopathy or broken heart syndrome. This condition is often triggered by intense emotional or physical stress, leading to transient left ventricular dysfunction. The hallmark of Takotsubo cardiomyopathy is the characteristic ballooning of the left ventricle's apex with basal hyperkinesis, resembling the shape of a Japanese octopus trap, known as a "takotsubo."

To confirm our suspicion, we performed a transthoracic echocardiogram. The echocardiographic images revealed apical ballooning of the left ventricle with hypercontractility of the basal segments, consistent with Takotsubo cardiomyopathy. The left ventricular ejection fraction (LVEF) was markedly reduced, measuring approximately 30%.

Laboratory investigations were carried out to support the diagnosis and rule out other potential causes. Cardiac biomarkers were elevated, particularly troponin I, indicative of myocardial injury. However, the levels were not as high as typically observed in extensive myocardial infarctions. Brain natriuretic peptide (BNP) was also elevated, suggesting increased ventricular stress and heart failure. Thyroid function tests, complete blood count, and a metabolic panel were within normal limits, excluding other potential contributors to the patient's condition.

With the diagnosis of Takotsubo cardiomyopathy established, we transitioned to the management phase. The cornerstone of treatment for this condition is supportive care, as the myocardial dysfunction is usually transient. The patient was admitted to the intensive care unit for close monitoring and management of hemodynamic status.

Initial management included the administration of aspirin and a statin, given the initial presentation mimicking an acute coronary syndrome. Beta-blockers and ACE inhibitors were initiated to support cardiac function and manage heart failure symptoms. The patient was started on metoprolol succinate 25 mg once daily and enalapril 5 mg once daily. Diuretics were administered to manage pulmonary congestion; furosemide 40 mg IV was given initially, followed by an oral dose of 20 mg twice daily.

Serial echocardiograms were performed to monitor the recovery of left ventricular function. Over the course of the first week, there was a gradual improvement in the LVEF, increasing to 40% by the seventh day. The patient's symptoms also showed significant improvement, with reduced chest pain and dyspnea.

To address the potential triggers, a thorough psychosocial assessment was conducted. The patient had experienced a recent bereavement, which likely precipitated the episode of Takotsubo cardiomyopathy. Psychological support and counseling were offered to help the patient cope with the emotional stress.

During the second week of hospitalization, the patient's condition continued to improve. The LVEF further increased to 50%, and the patient's functional status improved significantly. Diuretics were tapered off, and the doses of beta-blockers and ACE inhibitors were adjusted based on the patient's response and blood pressure.

Discharge planning involved comprehensive education on the nature of Takotsubo cardiomyopathy, its triggers, and the importance of medication adherence. The patient was prescribed metoprolol succinate 25 mg once daily and enalapril 5 mg once daily for continued outpatient management. A follow-up appointment with a cardiologist was scheduled for two weeks post-discharge to reassess cardiac function and adjust medications as necessary.

The patient was also referred to a psychologist for ongoing support to manage stress and prevent recurrence. Lifestyle modifications, including regular physical activity, a heart-healthy diet, and stress management techniques, were strongly recommended.

At the follow-up visit two weeks post-discharge, the patient's echocardiogram showed a near-complete resolution of the left ventricular dysfunction, with an LVEF of 60%. The patient remained asymptomatic, and their functional status had returned to baseline. Beta-blocker and ACE inhibitor therapy were continued, given their role in preventing recurrence and supporting long-term cardiac health.

In the third week following discharge, the patient

adhered to the prescribed medications and lifestyle recommendations. A comprehensive review of their daily activities and stress levels was conducted during follow-up visits. It was crucial to ensure that the patient avoided situations that could potentially trigger another episode of stress-induced cardiomyopathy.

Research indicates that Takotsubo cardiomyopathy predominantly affects postmenopausal women, but can also be seen in men and younger women. The pathophysiology involves a surge of catecholamines, such as adrenaline, in response to stress, which has a toxic effect on the myocardial cells, leading to stunning of the myocardium. This catecholamine surge can cause microvascular dysfunction and myocardial stunning, resulting in the characteristic apical ballooning seen on imaging studies.

The exact mechanisms by which catecholamines induce myocardial stunning in Takotsubo cardiomyopathy are not entirely understood, but several hypotheses have been proposed. These include direct myocardial toxicity, coronary artery spasm, microvascular dysfunction, and the effects of dynamic left ventricular outflow tract obstruction. The role of the sympathetic nervous system and the release of stress hormones are central to these hypotheses, linking emotional or physical stress to the onset of the syndrome.

Further follow-up at six weeks revealed sustained improvement. The patient's LVEF had normalized completely, measured at 65% on the latest echocardiogram. The patient's emotional well-being had also improved significantly with the support of psychological counseling and stress management strategies.

Despite the favorable outcome, it was imperative to educate the patient on the chronic nature of the condition and the possibility of recurrence. Patients with a history of Takotsubo cardiomyopathy should remain vigilant for symptoms of chest pain or dyspnea and seek immediate medical attention if such symptoms recur.

In terms of long-term prognosis, most patients recover completely within a few weeks to months, with normalization of left ventricular function. However, recurrence rates vary, with some studies suggesting recurrence in up to 10% of patients. Therefore, ongoing medical follow-up and management of cardiovascular risk factors are essential.

The multidisciplinary approach in this case was critical to the patient's recovery. Collaboration between cardiologists, primary care physicians, and mental health professionals ensured a holistic management plan. This case highlighted the importance of addressing not only the physiological aspects of the condition but also the psychological and emotional components.

The patient's journey through the diagnosis, treatment, and recovery of Takotsubo cardiomyopathy illustrated the complexities of managing stress-induced cardiac conditions.

❧ 7 ❧
FACTOR X DEFICIENCY

The case I'm about to describe is one of the most challenging and illuminating I've encountered in my career. It was a late autumn afternoon when the patient was admitted to the emergency department, presenting with unexplained bruising and prolonged bleeding from minor cuts. The patient's history indicated multiple episodes of spontaneous bleeding and excessive bleeding following dental procedures, which had been troubling for several years but had recently become more severe. Initial assessments did not suggest trauma or typical coagulation disorders, prompting a thorough investigation.

Upon physical examination, the patient had extensive ecchymosis on the arms and legs, without significant signs of trauma. Additionally, there was evidence of hemarthrosis in the right knee, causing noticeable swelling and discomfort. Basic blood tests were ordered, including a complete blood count (CBC), prothrombin time (PT), activated partial thromboplastin time (aPTT), and a comprehensive metabolic panel.

The results showed a normal platelet count and a mildly prolonged PT and aPTT. Given the normal platelet count, platelet function disorders were less likely. The mildly prolonged PT and aPTT suggested a problem with the common pathway of the coagulation cascade, pointing to potential deficiencies in factors V, X, or II, or the presence of an inhibitor.

Further specific factor assays were performed, which revealed significantly reduced activity of Factor X, at approximately 10% of normal levels. This finding was pivotal in diagnosing the patient with Factor X Deficiency, a rare autosomal recessive bleeding disorder. Factor X, also known as Stuart-Prower factor, is a vitamin K-dependent glycoprotein essential for the conversion of prothrombin to thrombin in the coagulation cascade.

Given the confirmed diagnosis, the next step was to develop an appropriate treatment plan. Factor X deficiency can range from mild to severe, with the patient exhibiting signs of a severe deficiency due to the extensive bleeding and low factor levels. The primary treatment goal was to control bleeding episodes and prevent future hemorrhages.

The treatment plan consisted of the following components:

- Replacement Therapy: The cornerstone of managing severe Factor X deficiency is replacement therapy. The patient was started on a regimen of prothrombin complex concentrates (PCCs), which contain Factors II, VII, IX, and X. The initial dose was calculated based on the patient's weight and the severity of the bleeding. An initial bolus of 30-50 units/kg of PCC was administered intravenously, followed by maintenance doses to maintain Factor X levels above 30% until the bleeding subsided.

- Fresh Frozen Plasma (FFP): In the absence of specific Factor X concentrates, FFP can be used as a source of Factor X. The patient received FFP in addition to PCC to provide a broader range of coagulation factors. This was particularly important during the initial phase of treatment to ensure adequate hemostasis.

- Vitamin K Supplementation: Since Factor X is a vitamin K-dependent protein, the patient was given vitamin K supplementation to optimize the synthesis of any residual Factor X. The patient received an initial dose of 10 mg of vitamin K intravenously, followed by daily oral doses to ensure adequate levels.

- Antifibrinolytic Agents: To further support hemostasis, the patient was given tranexamic acid, an antifibrinolytic agent that inhibits the breakdown of fibrin clots. This was particularly useful in managing mucosal bleeding and minor surgical procedures. The initial dose was 15 mg/kg intravenously, followed by oral doses of 1 gram three times daily for seven days.

- Monitoring and Follow-Up: Regular monitoring of Factor X levels and coagulation parameters was essential to adjust the treatment regimen as needed. The patient's PT and aPTT were checked daily initially, and Factor X levels were measured every other day. Liver function tests and vitamin K levels were also monitored to assess the patient's overall hemostatic status.

As the treatment progressed, the patient showed gradual improvement. The bleeding episodes decreased in frequency and severity, and the hemarthrosis resolved with supportive care and physiotherapy. After two weeks of intensive therapy, the patient's Factor X levels stabilized at around 20-30%, sufficient to prevent spontaneous bleeding.

Given the rarity of Factor X deficiency, genetic counseling was recommended for the patient and their family to discuss the inheritance patterns and implications for future offspring. The patient was also educated on recognizing early signs of bleeding and the importance of regular follow-up visits to monitor their condition.

Unfortunately, the chronic nature of severe Factor X deficiency meant that lifelong management was necessary. The patient was discharged with a comprehensive care plan, including home infusions of PCC for breakthrough bleeding episodes, oral vitamin K supplementation, and regular follow-ups at a specialized hematology clinic. The patient was also provided with an emergency card indicating their condition and treatment protocol in case of urgent medical situations.

Despite the chronic challenges, the patient's condition was stabilized, and they were able to return to a relatively normal life with appropriate medical support. The successful management of the patient's bleeding disorder through targeted replacement therapy, supportive care, and ongoing monitoring underscored the potential for improving quality of life even in rare and challenging medical conditions.

৺ 8 ঽ
ACDC

A s a medical practitioner with years of experience, I encountered numerous rare and complex cases. Among them, one stands out vividly in my memory—a case of Arterial Calcification Due to Deficiency of CD73 (ACDC). This rare genetic disorder, characterized by extensive calcium deposits in the arteries and joints, posed a significant diagnostic and therapeutic challenge.

☙❧

THE PATIENT, A MIDDLE-AGED INDIVIDUAL, CAME TO my clinic with complaints of severe pain and stiffness in the legs, particularly in the calves, thighs, and feet. The pain had progressively worsened over the past few years, severely impacting mobility. Walking had become a strenuous task, often accompanied by intense cramping and discomfort. Additionally, the patient reported noticeable deformities and stiffness in the fingers, making daily tasks increasingly difficult.

A thorough physical examination revealed several key findings. The arteries in the legs were palpably hardened, and there were irregular, bony nodules along the course of these vessels. The joints of the hands exhibited significant thickening and deformities, consistent with advanced calcification. Given these findings, a detailed diagnostic workup was warranted.

Initial blood tests were telling. The patient exhibited elevated levels of tissue-nonspecific alkaline phosphatase (TNAP) and reduced levels of pyrophosphate, a key inhibitor of calcium phosphate crystal formation. These biochemical markers strongly suggested a disorder of abnormal calcification. However, the definitive diagnosis required genetic analysis.

Genetic testing confirmed the presence of a mutation in the NT5E gene, responsible for encoding the CD73 enzyme. CD73 plays a crucial role in converting adenosine monophosphate to adenosine. In ACDC, this conversion is impaired due to the defective enzyme, leading to decreased adenosine levels. This deficiency, in turn, results in increased TNAP activity and decreased pyrophosphate levels, promoting the pathological calcification observed in the patient.

To further assess the extent of the calcification,

imaging studies were conducted. X-rays and CT angiography provided a clear picture of the severity. The arteries in the lower limbs were extensively calcified, creating significant stenosis and reducing blood flow. The joints of the hands showed advanced calcification, contributing to the patient's pain and deformity. These findings were consistent with the clinical and biochemical diagnosis of ACDC.

Given the rarity and severity of ACDC, the treatment plan had to be meticulously crafted. There was no known cure for the condition, and management primarily focused on alleviating symptoms and slowing disease progression. The cornerstone of the treatment was etidronate, a bisphosphonate that acts as a non-hydrolysable pyrophosphate analog. This drug had shown promise in clinical trials for inhibiting further calcification in ACDC patients.

The patient was prescribed etidronate at a dosage of 5 mg/kg/day for 14 days, to be repeated every three months. This intermittent dosing regimen aimed to balance efficacy with safety, minimizing potential side effects. Alongside etidronate, the patient was given anti-inflammatory medications to manage pain and inflammation. Physical therapy was also recommended to maintain joint mobility and muscle strength, crucial for preserving functional capacity.

Regular follow-up visits were essential to monitor the patient's response to treatment and adjust the plan as necessary. Annual CT scans were scheduled to track the progression of calcification in the arteries and joints. The ankle-brachial index, a non-invasive measure of blood flow, was used to assess vascular function in the lower limbs.

Over the course of three years, the patient's condition stabilized. The etidronate treatment effectively halted the progression of new calcification, as evidenced by the imaging studies. Pain levels, while still present, were better managed with the combination of anti-inflammatory medications and physical therapy. The patient reported improved mobility and a greater ability to perform daily activities, significantly enhancing the quality of life.

Despite these positive outcomes, it was important to acknowledge the limitations of the treatment. Etidronate did not reverse existing calcifications, and some degree of pain and stiffness persisted. However, the primary goal of preventing further deterioration was achieved, marking a significant success in managing this challenging condition.

Through a combination of targeted medication, supportive therapies, and regular monitoring, we were able to achieve significant improvements in the patient's condition, providing hope and a better quality of life amidst the challenges posed by this rare genetic disorder.

9

ACROOSTEOLYSIS DOMINANT TYPE

The patient, a 45-year-old male, presented to our clinic with complaints of chronic pain in the distal phalanges of his fingers and toes, accompanied by noticeable deformity. He reported a progressive worsening of symptoms over the past five years, including increasing difficulty in performing fine motor tasks and experiencing persistent skin ulcers that were slow to heal. His medical history was unremarkable, with no prior diagnoses of systemic diseases that could account for his symptoms. A thorough family history revealed that his father had experienced similar symptoms but was never formally diagnosed.

Upon physical examination, I observed significant swelling and deformity in the distal interphalangeal joints of the fingers and toes. There was also evidence of trophic changes in the skin, including atrophic, shiny skin, and several non-healing ulcers. The nails appeared dystrophic with onycholysis. Palpation revealed tenderness over the affected joints, but no significant warmth or erythema, suggesting a non-inflammatory process.

Given the presentation, a comprehensive diagnostic workup was initiated. Blood tests, including a complete blood count (CBC), erythrocyte sedimentation rate (ESR), C-reactive protein (CRP), and rheumatoid factor (RF), were ordered to rule out inflammatory and autoimmune etiologies. All results were within normal limits, except for a mildly elevated ESR, which was non-specific.

Radiographic imaging of the hands and feet was performed next. X-rays revealed marked resorption of the distal phalanges, characteristic of acroosteolysis. The resorption was most pronounced in the terminal tufts of the fingers and toes, with a 'penciling' appearance. There were no signs of periosteal reaction or new bone formation, which further supported the diagnosis of a non-inflammatory condition.

To confirm the diagnosis and exclude other differential diagnoses such as scleroderma, psoriatic arthritis, and primary hypertrophic osteoarthropathy, a genetic test was conducted. Sequencing of the MMP2 gene revealed a heterozygous mutation consistent with Acroosteolysis Dominant Type.

Based on the clinical presentation, radiographic findings, and genetic confirmation, the patient was diagnosed with Acroosteolysis Dominant Type. This rare genetic disorder, characterized by progressive bone resorption of the distal phalanges, often manifests in middle age and can lead to significant morbidity due to pain, deformity, and functional impairment.

Management of Acroosteolysis Dominant Type is challenging due to the progressive nature of the disease and the lack of curative treatment. The primary goals of treatment are to manage pain, prevent complications, and maintain function. The following multi-disciplinary treatment plan was developed:

1. Pain Management:

- Nonsteroidal Anti-inflammatory Drugs (NSAIDs): The patient was prescribed ibuprofen 800 mg three times daily to manage pain and reduce inflammation.
- Opioids: For breakthrough pain, a prescription for tramadol 50 mg as needed was provided, with careful monitoring to prevent dependency.
- Topical Analgesics: Capsaicin cream was recommended to be applied to affected areas to provide localized pain relief.

2. Bone Health:

- Bisphosphonates: Alendronate 70 mg once weekly was prescribed to slow down the bone resorption process. This was based on evidence suggesting bisphosphonates can be beneficial in reducing osteoclast-mediated bone resorption.

- Calcium and Vitamin D Supplementation: The patient was advised to take calcium 1000 mg and vitamin D 800 IU daily to support overall bone health.

3. Wound Care:

- Regular Dressing Changes: The patient was instructed on proper wound care techniques and scheduled for regular visits with a wound care specialist. Silver-impregnated dressings were used to promote healing and prevent infection.
- Antibiotics: In cases of infected ulcers, a course of oral antibiotics, such as cephalexin 500 mg four times daily for 10 days, was initiated.

4. Physical Therapy:

- A tailored physical therapy program was designed to maintain joint mobility and strengthen surrounding muscles. This included exercises to improve fine motor skills and prevent contractures.

5. Surgical Consultation:

- A referral to an orthopedic surgeon was made for evaluation of the possibility of surgical intervention to correct severe deformities and improve function. However, surgery was considered a last resort due to the risks associated with poor wound healing.

6. Genetic Counseling:

- The patient and his family were referred to a genetic counselor to discuss the hereditary nature of the condition and the implications for family planning and genetic testing for other family members.

The patient was closely monitored over the following months with regular follow-up visits every three months. During these visits, the patient's pain levels, functional status, and wound healing progress were assessed. Adjustments to the treatment plan were made based on the patient's response to therapy.

In the initial three-month follow-up, the patient reported a modest reduction in pain levels with the use of NSAIDs and tramadol. The capsaicin cream provided some relief for localized pain. However, the non-healing ulcers remained a significant concern. Despite regular wound care and antibiotic treatment, the ulcers showed minimal improvement.

Radiographic imaging at this stage did not reveal any significant progression of bone resorption, indicating that the bisphosphonate therapy might be exerting a stabilizing effect. Physical therapy sessions helped the patient maintain joint mobility, though fine motor skills remained impaired.

At the six-month follow-up, the patient's condition had not significantly improved. Pain management remained a challenge, with increasing reliance on tramadol for breakthrough pain. The patient expressed frustration with the chronic nature of the condition and the limited effectiveness of the current treatment regimen.

Wound care continued to be problematic, with recurrent infections requiring multiple courses of antibiotics. Despite aggressive wound management, some ulcers progressed to deeper infections, necessitating surgical debridement. The orthopedic surgeon advised against corrective surgery for deformities due to the high risk of complications.

At the one-year follow-up, the patient's condition had deteriorated further. The chronic pain and functional impairment significantly affected his quality of life. The distal phalanges continued to resorb, leading to increasing deformity and disability. The persistent skin ulcers led to recurrent infections, some of which resulted in osteomyelitis.

Despite the multi-disciplinary approach and aggressive management, the patient's overall prognosis remained poor. The progressive nature of Acroosteolysis Dominant Type, coupled with the lack of effective treatments to halt or reverse bone resorption, posed significant challenges.

Ultimately, the patient succumbed to complications related to chronic infections and sepsis. The recurrent osteomyelitis, coupled with systemic infection, proved fatal. This case highlights the severe impact of Acroosteolysis Dominant Type and underscores the need for further research into effective treatments and management strategies for this debilitating condition.

ACROOSTEOLYSIS DOMINANT TYPE IS A RARE GENETIC disorder characterized by progressive resorption of the distal phalanges, leading to significant pain, deformity, and functional impairment. Despite current treatment modalities aimed at managing symptoms and preventing complications, the prognosis remains poor due to the relentless progression of the disease and the lack of curative options.

10

ACUTE MONOBLASTIC LEUKEMIA

The patient presented to the clinic with symptoms that had progressively worsened over the past several weeks. The initial complaints were fatigue, bruising, and occasional nosebleeds. Upon physical examination, pallor and petechiae were noted, indicative of possible hematologic abnormalities. Given the constellation of symptoms, I immediately ordered a complete blood count (CBC) and peripheral blood smear.

The CBC revealed pancytopenia with a significantly elevated white blood cell (WBC) count. The differential showed a predominance of monoblasts. The hemoglobin was critically low at 7.2 g/dL, and the platelet count was 32,000/µL, well below the normal range. These findings suggested a possible acute leukemia, specifically a type involving monoblasts. I proceeded with a bone marrow biopsy and aspirate to confirm the diagnosis and assess the extent of marrow infiltration.

The bone marrow aspirate was hypercellular with over 80% monoblasts. Flow cytometry analysis of the bone marrow confirmed the diagnosis of Acute Monoblastic Leukemia (AML-M5), characterized by the presence of CD13, CD33, CD14, CD4, and CD11b markers. Cytogenetic analysis revealed a translocation involving chromosomes 9 and 11 [t(9;11)(p22;q23)], commonly associated with this leukemia subtype.

With the diagnosis confirmed, I promptly initiated the treatment plan. Given the aggressive nature of Acute Monoblastic Leukemia, immediate hospitalization was necessary. The patient was admitted to the oncology unit, where we began induction chemotherapy using the standard "7+3" regimen: seven days of continuous infusion of cytarabine (100 mg/m²/day) combined with three days of daunorubicin (60 mg/m²/day).

The first week of chemotherapy was intense. Cytarabine, an antimetabolite, works by interfering with DNA synthesis, targeting rapidly dividing cells such as the leukemic blasts. Daunorubicin, an anthracycline, intercalates into DNA and inhibits topoisomerase II, causing breaks in DNA strands and inducing apoptosis in cancer cells. Throughout the treatment, the patient was monitored closely for side effects, including myelosuppression, mucositis, and the risk of infections due to neutropenia.

Supportive care played a crucial role in managing the

complications of chemotherapy. The patient received prophylactic antibiotics, antifungals, and antivirals to prevent opportunistic infections. Additionally, transfusions of packed red blood cells and platelets were administered to manage anemia and thrombocytopenia. The patient also received granulocyte colony-stimulating factor (G-CSF) to stimulate the production of neutrophils and reduce the duration of neutropenia.

After completing the induction phase, a repeat bone marrow biopsy was performed to assess the response to treatment. Unfortunately, the biopsy revealed persistent disease with 20% residual blasts. This indicated that the patient had not achieved complete remission, and a second round of induction chemotherapy was necessary. The re-induction regimen consisted of high-dose cytarabine (HiDAC) and mitoxantrone, another anthracycline similar to daunorubicin but with a different toxicity profile.

The second induction was more grueling. The high-dose cytarabine regimen significantly increased the risk of neurotoxicity and cytopenias. The patient developed severe mucositis, making oral intake difficult, necessitating parenteral nutrition and intensive pain management. Despite these challenges, the patient remained resilient, and after the second cycle, the bone marrow biopsy showed a marked reduction in blast cells to less than 5%, indicating a partial remission.

Given the partial remission, it was essential to

consolidate the response and prevent relapse. The patient underwent consolidation chemotherapy with intermediate-dose cytarabine over three cycles. Each cycle involved the administration of cytarabine over five days every four weeks. This phase aimed to eradicate any residual leukemic cells and secure long-term remission.

Throughout the consolidation phase, the patient experienced multiple complications. Episodes of febrile neutropenia required frequent hospitalizations, broad-spectrum antibiotics, and antifungal therapy. The patient also developed hemorrhagic cystitis, a known side effect of cytarabine, which was managed with aggressive hydration and continuous bladder irrigation.

With the completion of consolidation chemotherapy, the patient achieved complete remission. However, the high risk of relapse associated with AML-M5, particularly with the t(9;11) translocation, necessitated consideration of a hematopoietic stem cell transplant (HSCT). After a thorough evaluation, the patient was deemed a suitable candidate for an allogeneic HSCT, given the presence of a matched sibling donor.

The preparative regimen for HSCT consisted of a myeloablative conditioning regimen with busulfan and cyclophosphamide. Busulfan was administered over four days, followed by cyclophosphamide for two days, to eradicate the patient's bone marrow and create space for the donor stem cells. This regimen was chosen for its efficacy in achieving long-term disease control in AML patients.

The transplantation procedure itself went smoothly. The donor stem cells were infused intravenously, and engraftment was monitored through daily blood counts and chimerism studies. Engraftment occurred on day 15 post-transplant, marked by a rising neutrophil count and donor-derived hematopoiesis. The patient was monitored for graft-versus-host disease (GVHD), a common complication where the donor immune cells attack the recipient's tissues. Prophylactic immunosuppressive therapy with tacrolimus and methotrexate was initiated to mitigate this risk.

Despite the prophylactic measures, the patient developed acute GVHD affecting the skin and gastrointestinal tract. The skin involvement presented as a maculopapular rash, while the gastrointestinal symptoms included diarrhea and abdominal pain. High-dose corticosteroids were administered to control the GVHD, and the patient responded well, with gradual resolution of symptoms.

Over the following months, the patient remained in remission and continued to recover from the transplant. Regular follow-ups included bone marrow biopsies and molecular studies to monitor for minimal residual disease (MRD). Fortunately, all tests remained negative, indicating sustained remission.

As part of the long-term follow-up, the patient was

monitored for late complications of HSCT, such as chronic GVHD, infections, and secondary malignancies. Regular vaccinations and prophylactic antibiotics were essential to prevent infections, given the long-term immunosuppression.

The patient's journey through the diagnosis and treatment of Acute Monoblastic Leukemia was arduous, marked by numerous challenges and complications. However, through aggressive treatment, supportive care, and the successful hematopoietic stem cell transplant, the patient achieved and maintained complete remission.

✾ 11 ✾

ALIEN HAND SYNDROME

The patient was a middle-aged individual, presenting with a peculiar and distressing condition that had perplexed several physicians before reaching my clinic. They arrived with complaints of involuntary hand movements, specifically the left hand, which seemed to act with a mind of its own. Upon initial observation, the patient's left hand frequently engaged in unintentional actions such as buttoning and unbuttoning their shirt, grabbing objects without conscious intent, and even slapping themselves. These movements were often counterproductive to the patient's conscious efforts with their right hand, creating a scenario of internal conflict and frustration.

Upon thorough history taking, the patient revealed that these symptoms had gradually developed over the past few months. There was no significant trauma reported to the head or limbs, but the patient did have a history of cerebrovascular accidents (CVA) and reported a transient ischemic attack (TIA) approximately a year prior. This provided a crucial lead as Alien Hand Syndrome (AHS) is often associated with lesions in the corpus callosum, frontal lobes, or parietal lobes—regions commonly affected by strokes.

To confirm the diagnosis, a detailed neurological examination was conducted. The patient demonstrated normal strength and coordination in the right hand, but the left hand exhibited autonomous movements without the patient's awareness. This disassociation between conscious intent and action was a hallmark of AHS. The patient also reported a lack of proprioceptive feedback from the affected hand, further substantiating the diagnosis. Cognitive function tests showed no significant impairment, ruling out other neuropsychiatric conditions.

Magnetic Resonance Imaging (MRI) of the brain was ordered to identify any structural anomalies. The imaging revealed a lesion in the corpus callosum, specifically in the anterior portion, which corroborated the clinical findings. The corpus callosum is a major cerebral commissure that facilitates interhemispheric communication. Damage to this structure disrupts the coordination between the hemispheres, leading to the manifestation of AHS.

Given the confirmation of Alien Hand Syndrome, the

treatment plan needed to be multifaceted, focusing on both symptom management and rehabilitation. The primary goal was to mitigate the disruptive actions of the alien hand and improve the patient's quality of life.

First, pharmacological intervention was considered. Clonazepam, a benzodiazepine, was prescribed at a dose of 0.5 mg twice daily. Benzodiazepines are known for their muscle relaxant properties and can help reduce involuntary movements. Additionally, a low dose of botulinum toxin was injected into the overactive muscles of the left hand. Botulinum toxin works by inhibiting acetylcholine release at the neuromuscular junction, thus reducing muscle contractions and the severity of involuntary movements.

Parallel to pharmacological treatment, occupational therapy was initiated. The patient was enrolled in a specialized rehabilitation program that included constraint-induced movement therapy (CIMT). In this approach, the unaffected hand was constrained to encourage the use of the affected hand under controlled circumstances. This therapy aimed to improve the neural plasticity and functional integration of the alien hand into purposeful actions. Regular sessions were scheduled to monitor progress and adjust techniques as necessary.

Behavioral strategies were also introduced. The patient was taught to use visual and tactile cues to regain control over the alien hand. For instance, wearing a glove on the affected hand provided sensory feedback and served as a reminder of its position and actions. Engaging the alien hand in purposeful activities, like holding an object or performing repetitive tasks, helped in reducing its erratic behavior.

In addition to these interventions, psychological support was provided. Alien Hand Syndrome can be a distressing condition, leading to anxiety and depression. Regular counseling sessions were arranged to help the patient cope with the psychological impact of the disorder. Cognitive-behavioral therapy (CBT) was particularly effective in addressing the patient's feelings of helplessness and frustration, fostering a positive outlook towards the rehabilitation process.

Follow-up appointments were scheduled at regular intervals to assess the efficacy of the treatment plan. Over the next few months, the patient showed gradual improvement. The frequency and intensity of the involuntary movements decreased significantly. The patient reported better control over the alien hand, with fewer instances of disruptive behavior. Occupational therapy sessions were particularly beneficial in enhancing the functional integration of the alien hand.

Despite these improvements, the condition persisted, albeit at a reduced severity. Alien Hand Syndrome is a chronic condition with no definitive cure. The goal of treatment was to manage symptoms and improve the patient's quality of life. The patient continued to use behavioral strategies and pharmacological support to maintain control over the alien hand.

Throughout the course of treatment, the patient remained motivated and compliant with the therapeutic regimen. Their resilience and determination played a crucial role in the overall management of the condition. Regular assessments and adjustments to the treatment plan ensured that the interventions remained effective and relevant to the patient's needs.

In summary, the patient's case of Alien Hand Syndrome was successfully managed through a comprehensive approach involving pharmacological treatment, occupational therapy, behavioral strategies, and psychological support. While the condition could not be completely eradicated, significant improvements in symptom control and quality of life were achieved.

AMYOTROPHIC LATERAL SCLEROSIS
TYPE 7

I first encountered the patient during a routine neurological consultation. A middle-aged individual, they presented with progressively worsening weakness, primarily in the distal muscles of the hands and legs. This weakness had been developing insidiously over several months, and the patient also reported occasional muscle cramps and twitching, particularly in the forearms and calves. As I took their history, it became evident that these symptoms were steadily advancing, significantly impacting their ability to perform daily tasks such as buttoning shirts, opening jars, and walking without tripping.

Upon conducting a thorough physical examination, I noted several hallmark features of a motor neuron disease. The patient exhibited significant muscle atrophy in the thenar and hypothenar eminences of the hands, as well as in the tibialis anterior muscles of the legs. Fasciculations, or muscle twitches, were visible beneath the skin, particularly in the aforementioned areas. Reflexes were brisk, especially in the limbs, and the Babinski sign was positive bilaterally, indicating upper motor neuron involvement. Additionally, I observed that the patient's gait was spastic and their speech was slightly slurred, suggesting bulbar involvement.

Given the combination of upper and lower motor neuron signs, my differential diagnosis narrowed considerably. Amyotrophic lateral sclerosis (ALS) was at the forefront of my considerations, and the specific variant, ALS type 7, which involves mutations in the SOD1 gene, seemed a likely candidate given the patient's age and symptomatology. I explained the need for further diagnostic workup, including electromyography (EMG), nerve conduction studies (NCS), and genetic testing.

The EMG revealed widespread denervation and reinnervation changes in the limbs, indicative of ongoing neurogenic atrophy and compensatory sprouting by surviving motor neurons. The NCS showed normal sensory nerve action potentials, ruling out a primary sensory neuropathy, but there was reduced compound muscle action potential amplitude, consistent with motor axon loss. Genetic testing confirmed a mutation in the SOD1 gene, specifically a p.A4V substitution, which is known to be associated with a rapidly progressive form of ALS.

With the diagnosis of ALS type 7 confirmed, I outlined a comprehensive treatment plan aimed at managing symptoms and maintaining quality of life, as there is no cure for ALS. Riluzole, a glutamate inhibitor, was prescribed to slow disease progression. This medication has been shown to extend survival modestly by reducing excitotoxic damage to motor neurons. The patient was instructed to take 50 mg twice daily, and liver function tests were scheduled periodically to monitor for potential hepatotoxicity.

In addition to pharmacological treatment, I emphasized the importance of multidisciplinary care. A referral was made to a specialized ALS clinic where the patient could receive coordinated care from neurologists, physical therapists, occupational therapists, speech and language therapists, and nutritionists. This team approach is essential in managing the diverse and progressive challenges of ALS.

Physical therapy focused on maintaining strength and flexibility, with a tailored exercise program to prevent contractures and joint stiffness. Occupational therapy provided adaptive equipment to assist with activities of daily living, such as eating, dressing, and personal hygiene. Speech and language therapy was initiated early to address dysarthria and dysphagia, which are common as the disease progresses. A dietitian provided guidance on maintaining adequate nutrition, emphasizing the importance of a high-calorie diet to combat the hyper-metabolic state often seen in ALS patients.

As the disease advanced, respiratory function became a critical aspect of care. Regular pulmonary function tests were conducted to monitor vital capacity and detect any decline in respiratory muscle strength. Non-invasive ventilation (NIV) was introduced when the patient's forced vital capacity dropped below 50% of the predicted value, or earlier if they experienced symptoms of nocturnal hypoventilation, such as morning headaches, fatigue, or dyspnea. NIV, using a bilevel positive airway pressure (BiPAP) machine, can significantly improve quality of life and survival in ALS patients by providing respiratory support and reducing the work of breathing.

As swallowing difficulties progressed, the risk of aspiration and malnutrition increased. The patient was evaluated for a percutaneous endoscopic gastrostomy (PEG) tube placement to ensure adequate nutrition and hydration while minimizing the risk of aspiration pneumonia. PEG placement is typically recommended when the patient's weight loss exceeds 10% of their baseline body weight, or when swallowing difficulties severely impact oral intake.

Throughout the course of the disease, I closely monitored the patient's progression using the ALS Functional Rating Scale-Revised (ALSFRS-R), which assesses the patient's ability to perform daily activities and their respiratory function. This tool helped to guide clinical decisions and adjust the care plan as needed.

As the patient's condition deteriorated, palliative care and hospice services became integral to their management. Palliative care focused on symptom relief, addressing issues such as pain, dyspnea, anxiety, and depression. A combination of medications, including opioids for pain and dyspnea, anxiolytics for anxiety, and antidepressants for mood disturbances, was used to manage these symptoms effectively. Hospice care provided support not only for the patient but also for their family, offering emotional and psychological support during this difficult time.

Despite the comprehensive and multidisciplinary approach to care, ALS type 7 is relentlessly progressive. The patient eventually developed significant bulbar involvement, characterized by severe dysarthria, dysphagia, and emotional lability. Respiratory failure became the primary concern, and despite the use of NIV, the patient's respiratory muscles weakened to the point where they could no longer maintain adequate ventilation.

After extensive discussions with the patient and their family about their goals of care and end-of-life wishes, it was decided to focus on comfort measures. The patient was transitioned to hospice care, where the emphasis was placed on providing comfort and dignity in their final days. Medications were adjusted to prioritize symptom control, and the patient was surrounded by their loved ones.

In the final stages, managing the patient's symptoms required a delicate balance of medications. Opioids were titrated to manage pain and dyspnea effectively without causing excessive sedation. Anxiolytics were used to alleviate the patient's anxiety and restlessness, which often accompany respiratory distress. Anticholinergic medications helped reduce the excessive salivation and secretions that are common in ALS, which can exacerbate choking and aspiration risks.

Throughout this period, I maintained close communication with the hospice team to ensure the patient's comfort and address any emerging symptoms promptly. The focus was on providing holistic care that encompassed not only physical symptoms but also emotional and psychological support for both the patient and their family. The hospice team included counselors and social workers who provided invaluable support, helping the family cope with the impending loss and navigate the complexities of end-of-life care.

The patient's decline was marked by increasing fatigue and sleepiness, as respiratory muscles failed to support adequate gas exchange even with NIV assistance. The decision was made to discontinue NIV when it no longer provided meaningful relief and only served to prolong discomfort. The patient was transitioned to a regimen of continuous oxygen therapy and medication adjustments aimed at ensuring a peaceful and dignified passing.

The patient's final days were spent in a tranquil environment, free from the invasive interventions that had characterized earlier stages of the disease. Pain and anxiety were well-controlled, allowing the patient to experience as much comfort as possible. The hospice team provided continuous care, ensuring that the patient's needs were met promptly and compassionately.

The patient passed away peacefully a few weeks later, succumbing to respiratory failure, which is the most common cause of death in ALS patients. Their death underscored the devastating nature of ALS and the need for ongoing research to find more effective treatments and ultimately a cure.

In the aftermath of the patient's passing, I reviewed the course of their disease and the care provided. The progression from initial symptoms to the terminal phase was swift, consistent with the aggressive nature of ALS type 7. Each stage presented unique challenges that required tailored interventions and vigilant monitoring. The collaboration among the multidisciplinary team was crucial in addressing the diverse needs of the patient, from mobility aids and nutritional support to respiratory management and end-of-life care.

The genetic basis of ALS type 7, specifically the SOD1 mutation, highlighted the importance of genetic counseling for the patient's family. Given the hereditary nature of this form of ALS, family members were offered genetic testing and counseling to understand their risks and potential implications for their health. This aspect of care extended beyond the patient, aiming to provide clarity and support to those who might be affected by the genetic predisposition.

❧ 13 ❧

ZUSKA'S DISEASE

The patient first presented to my clinic with a complaint of recurring abscesses in the subareolar region of her breasts. She was a 34-year-old woman with no significant past medical history. Upon examination, I noted induration and erythema in the affected areas, accompanied by intermittent purulent discharge. These symptoms were consistent with Zuska's disease, a rare chronic condition also known as periductal mastitis.

To confirm the diagnosis, I ordered an ultrasound of the breast, which revealed dilated ducts with periductal inflammation. Additionally, I requested a mammogram to rule out malignancy, which fortunately showed no signs of cancer. A swab of the purulent discharge was taken for culture and sensitivity testing to identify any bacterial pathogens present.

The pathogenesis of Zuska's disease involves the inflammation and infection of the mammary ducts, typically associated with smoking. However, our patient was a non-smoker, which made her case atypical. Nonetheless, the clinical presentation and imaging findings were unmistakable.

The primary goal of treatment was to alleviate symptoms and prevent recurrence. I initiated a course of broad-spectrum antibiotics, specifically amoxicillin-clavulanate, to address the bacterial infection identified in the culture results. The patient was advised to complete the entire course of antibiotics, even if symptoms improved earlier, to prevent the development of antibiotic-resistant bacteria.

Given the chronic nature of Zuska's disease and its tendency to recur, I also prescribed a topical steroid cream to reduce inflammation and pain. The patient was instructed to apply the cream twice daily to the affected areas. In addition, I recommended warm compresses to aid in the drainage of abscesses and promote healing.

To address the underlying issue of ductal obstruction, I referred the patient to a breast surgeon for further evaluation. Surgical intervention is often required in cases where conservative treatment fails to provide long-term relief. The surgical options included duct excision or, in more severe cases, total ductal excision.

During her follow-up visit two weeks later, the patient reported significant improvement in her symptoms. The erythema had decreased, and the discharge was minimal. The culture results had indicated a mixed infection with Staphylococcus aureus and anaerobic bacteria, which the prescribed antibiotics effectively targeted.

Despite the initial improvement, I emphasized the importance of maintaining vigilant breast hygiene and monitoring for any signs of recurrence. I also discussed the potential need for surgical intervention if symptoms persisted or recurred. The patient was receptive to the information and committed to following the treatment plan.

Over the next few months, the patient experienced intermittent flare-ups, characterized by mild pain and minimal discharge. Each episode was managed with short courses of antibiotics and continued use of the topical steroid cream. However, the frequency of these flare-ups gradually decreased, indicating a positive response to the ongoing treatment.

Six months into the treatment, the patient reported her longest period of remission since the onset of her symptoms. She had not experienced any significant flare-ups for nearly two months. On examination, the subareolar regions appeared normal, with no signs of inflammation or discharge. The patient expressed relief and satisfaction with the progress made.

At this point, we discussed the possibility of tapering off the topical steroid cream to avoid potential side effects associated with long-term use. The patient was instructed to gradually reduce the frequency of application over the next few weeks while continuing to monitor for any signs of recurrence. Additionally, I reinforced the importance of regular breast self-examinations and follow-up appointments to ensure ongoing monitoring and prompt intervention if needed.

In the subsequent months, the patient remained symptom-free. During her one-year follow-up visit, she expressed gratitude for the comprehensive care provided and reported a significant improvement in her quality of life. The absence of recurrent infections and the successful management of her symptoms marked a positive outcome for this case of Zuska's disease.

The integration of pharmacological and non-pharmacological treatments, along with patient education and adherence to the treatment plan, was instrumental in achieving long-term remission.

The patient responded well to the combination of antibiotic therapy, topical steroids, and supportive measures. Although the disease can be challenging to manage due to its chronic and recurrent nature, early diagnosis, appropriate treatment, and regular follow-up can significantly improve patient outcomes.

WILSON DISEASE

Wilson disease is a rare genetic disorder that leads to excessive accumulation of copper in the body. As a doctor with a keen interest in rare diseases, I had the opportunity to treat a patient who presented with this condition. This case stands out in my memory due to its complexity and the profound impact it had on my understanding of the disease.

THE PATIENT WAS A 32-YEAR-OLD MALE WHO ARRIVED at the clinic with a constellation of symptoms that had progressively worsened over the past several months. He had been experiencing fatigue, abdominal pain, and joint pain. Over time, he developed neuropsychiatric symptoms, including tremors, difficulty with speech, and mood changes. His family had noticed a significant alteration in his personality, with increased irritability and bouts of depression.

On initial examination, the patient appeared jaundiced with a slight greenish tint to his sclerae. His abdomen was distended, and he exhibited tenderness in the right upper quadrant. Neurological examination revealed dysarthria, asterixis, and a resting tremor. He also had mild hepatosplenomegaly, which was confirmed on palpation. These findings prompted me to consider a hepatic or metabolic disorder as the underlying cause.

Given the patient's presentation, I ordered a comprehensive set of laboratory tests. The initial blood work revealed elevated liver enzymes, particularly aspartate aminotransferase (AST) and alanine aminotransferase (ALT). The patient's bilirubin levels were also elevated, consistent with his jaundiced appearance. His serum ceruloplasmin level was notably low, at 10 mg/dL (normal range: 20-35 mg/dL). This finding raised my suspicion for Wilson disease, as ceruloplasmin is a copper-carrying protein in the blood, and low levels are a hallmark of the disorder.

To confirm the diagnosis, I requested a 24-hour urinary copper excretion test, which showed markedly elevated copper levels at 1500 µg (normal range: 15-60 µg). Additionally, a slit-lamp examination revealed the presence of Kayser-Fleischer rings, brownish or greenish rings around the cornea caused by copper deposition. These findings, combined with the clinical presentation and laboratory results, confirmed the diagnosis of Wilson disease.

Wilson disease is an autosomal recessive disorder caused by mutations in the ATP7B gene, which encodes a protein responsible for copper transport in the liver. In affected individuals, copper is not properly excreted into bile and instead accumulates in the liver, brain, and other tissues, leading to hepatocellular damage and neurological symptoms.

The primary goal of treatment for Wilson disease is to reduce copper levels in the body and prevent further accumulation. The treatment plan I devised for the patient involved several key components: chelation therapy, zinc supplementation, dietary modifications, and regular monitoring.

Chelation therapy is the cornerstone of treatment for Wilson disease. Chelating agents bind to copper, allowing it to be excreted in the urine. I prescribed penicillamine, an effective chelator, at a dose of 250 mg four times daily. Penicillamine can cause side effects such as hypersensitivity reactions, bone marrow suppression, and nephrotoxicity, so I closely monitored the patient for any adverse effects.

In addition to chelation therapy, I prescribed zinc acetate, which inhibits the absorption of copper from the gastrointestinal tract. The patient was instructed to take 50 mg of elemental zinc three times daily on an empty stomach. Zinc therapy can cause gastrointestinal discomfort, but it is generally well-tolerated and is an important adjunct to chelation therapy.

Dietary modifications were also necessary to reduce copper intake. I advised the patient to avoid foods high in copper, such as shellfish, nuts, chocolate, and organ meats. I provided a detailed list of foods to avoid and recommended consulting with a dietitian to develop a balanced, copper-restricted diet.

Regular monitoring was essential to assess the effectiveness of treatment and adjust the regimen as needed. I scheduled follow-up appointments every three months to monitor the patient's liver function tests, serum ceruloplasmin levels, and 24-hour urinary copper excretion. We also monitored the patient for any signs of treatment-related toxicity and made adjustments as necessary.

Over the next several months, the patient's condition began to improve. His liver enzyme levels gradually normalized, and his bilirubin levels decreased. The neurological symptoms, while slow to resolve, showed signs of improvement as well. The tremors and dysarthria lessened, and his mood stabilized. The patient adhered well to the treatment regimen, and we continued to adjust the dosages based on his response and laboratory results.

However, the road to recovery was not without challenges. The patient experienced episodes of gastrointestinal discomfort due to the zinc supplementation, and we had to adjust the timing and dosage to minimize these side effects. Additionally, penicillamine caused mild leucopenia, necessitating a temporary reduction in the dose and close monitoring of his blood counts.

Despite these setbacks, the patient's overall trajectory was positive. By the end of the first year of treatment, his liver function tests were within normal limits, and his urinary copper excretion had decreased significantly, indicating effective copper chelation. His neurological symptoms had largely resolved, although he still experienced occasional tremors and fatigue.

Throughout the treatment process, I emphasized the importance of lifelong adherence to the treatment regimen and regular follow-up. Wilson disease requires ongoing management to prevent copper reaccumulation and long-term complications. The patient was educated about the chronic nature of the disease and the necessity of continuous monitoring and treatment.

In the second year of treatment, the patient continued to show improvement. His liver function remained stable, and his neuropsychiatric symptoms were well-controlled. He had adapted to the dietary restrictions and incorporated them into his lifestyle. The patient's quality of life had significantly improved, and he was able to resume many of his daily activities and work responsibilities.

However, it is important to note that Wilson disease

can have a variable prognosis depending on the severity of liver and neurological involvement at the time of diagnosis. Early detection and initiation of treatment are crucial for a favorable outcome. In cases where significant liver damage has occurred, liver transplantation may be necessary. Fortunately, in this patient's case, the timely diagnosis and initiation of treatment allowed for a good recovery without the need for transplantation.

By the end of the third year, the patient's condition had stabilized, and he was in remission. His liver function tests remained normal, and his urinary copper excretion was well-controlled. He continued to take penicillamine and zinc as prescribed and adhered to his dietary restrictions. Regular follow-up appointments were scheduled every six months to monitor his condition and adjust treatment as necessary.

❧ 15 ❧

VASCULAR HYALINOSIS

I remember the patient as clearly as any other who has left a significant mark on my medical career. The case was a striking example of the challenges posed by vascular hyalinosis, a condition often encountered but seldom understood in its full complexity.

❧

THE PATIENT PRESENTED WITH SYMPTOMS THAT WERE initially vague and non-specific: general fatigue, mild dizziness, and occasional headaches. These complaints could easily be attributed to a variety of common conditions. However, a closer examination revealed telltale signs that hinted at something more serious. The patient's blood pressure was consistently elevated, registering at 160/100 mmHg during the initial consultation.

Additionally, there was mild proteinuria detected in a routine urinalysis, suggesting a potential renal involvement.

I proceeded with a thorough clinical evaluation. The patient was in their late 60s, had a history of poorly controlled hypertension, and was a long-term smoker, all of which are significant risk factors for vascular disease. Physical examination showed no acute distress, but there were subtle signs such as decreased peripheral pulses and slight edema in the lower extremities.

Given the patient's history and the clinical findings, I ordered a series of diagnostic tests. A comprehensive metabolic panel was conducted, revealing elevated serum creatinine levels of 1.8 mg/dL, indicating compromised renal function. An ECG showed left ventricular hypertrophy, consistent with the prolonged hypertension. Most crucially, a renal ultrasound demonstrated small, echogenic kidneys, which are characteristic of chronic hypertensive nephropathy.

To confirm the diagnosis and assess the extent of vascular damage, I decided to perform a renal biopsy. The histopathological examination of the biopsy samples provided definitive evidence. There was marked hyalinosis in the afferent arterioles, with homogenous, eosinophilic deposits of hyaline material observed in the vessel walls. These changes were indicative of chronic damage due to persistent hypertension, leading to ischemia and subsequent fibrosis in the kidney tissue.

The glomeruli showed segmental sclerosis, and there was moderate interstitial fibrosis and tubular atrophy.

The diagnosis was confirmed: the patient had vascular hyalinosis, a condition characterized by the deposition of hyaline material in the walls of small arteries and arterioles, leading to luminal narrowing and reduced blood flow. This pathology was primarily a consequence of long-standing hypertension, compounded by the patient's smoking history.

With the diagnosis in hand, the next step was to formulate a comprehensive treatment plan. The primary goal was to manage the patient's hypertension more effectively to prevent further vascular and renal damage. I prescribed a combination of antihypertensive medications: an angiotensin-converting enzyme (ACE) inhibitor, lisinopril, at a dose of 10 mg daily, to reduce blood pressure and provide renal protection; a calcium channel blocker, amlodipine, at 5 mg daily, to help control blood pressure; and a diuretic, hydrochlorothiazide, at 25 mg daily, to manage fluid retention and further aid in blood pressure control.

In addition to pharmacotherapy, I emphasized the importance of lifestyle modifications. The patient was advised to quit smoking immediately, as continued tobacco use would exacerbate vascular damage. I referred them to a smoking cessation program to increase the chances of success. Dietary changes were also recommended, including a low-sodium diet to help control blood pressure and a renal-friendly diet to reduce the burden on the kidneys. Regular physical activity, tailored to the patient's abilities and health status, was encouraged to improve cardiovascular health.

Regular follow-up appointments were scheduled to monitor the patient's progress. Blood pressure was checked at each visit, and adjustments to the medication regimen were made as necessary to achieve optimal control. Repeat laboratory tests, including serum creatinine and urinalysis, were performed periodically to assess renal function. Over the next several months, the patient's blood pressure gradually came under control, with readings consistently below 140/90 mmHg.

Despite these efforts, the chronic nature of vascular hyalinosis meant that complete reversal of the damage was not possible. However, the goal was to prevent further progression of the disease. During the follow-up period, the patient's renal function remained stable, with serum creatinine levels fluctuating around 1.8-2.0 mg/dL. Proteinuria persisted but did not worsen significantly. The patient reported an overall improvement in symptoms, with reduced dizziness and headaches, and a modest increase in energy levels.

Unfortunately, the long-term prognosis for patients with vascular hyalinosis is guarded. While we were able to stabilize the patient's condition and prevent acute deterioration, the underlying vascular damage continued to pose a risk for future complications. Over the course of two years, the patient experienced a gradual decline in renal function, with serum creatinine rising to 2.5 mg/dL, indicating worsening chronic kidney disease. Despite this, the patient remained compliant with the treatment plan and continued to follow the recommended lifestyle modifications.

In the end, the patient succumbed to the complications associated with advanced vascular disease. A severe hypertensive crisis led to acute renal failure and subsequently to multi-organ failure. Despite aggressive medical intervention, the damage was too extensive to reverse. The patient passed away peacefully in the hospital, surrounded by family.

While the outcome was ultimately fatal, the interventions provided extended the patient's life and improved the quality of the remaining years.

UNVERRICHT-LUNDBORG DISEASE

The patient was a 19-year-old male who presented to my neurology clinic with a chief complaint of frequent myoclonic jerks and increasing difficulty with coordination. His symptoms had begun insidiously around the age of 15, with occasional muscle twitches that were initially sporadic and easily ignored. Over the past year, however, these twitches had progressed to more frequent and severe myoclonic jerks, often causing him to drop objects or fall. Additionally, he reported a progressive decline in his coordination and balance, making daily activities increasingly challenging.

Upon examination, the patient exhibited frequent, spontaneous myoclonic jerks predominantly affecting his upper limbs. These jerks were exacerbated by voluntary movement and emotional stress. His gait was ataxic, characterized by unsteady, wide-based steps, and he required assistance to walk. The neurological examination revealed dysmetria, evident through a positive finger-to-nose test, and intention tremor. He also displayed dysarthria, with slurred and slow speech. There was no evidence of muscle weakness or sensory deficits, but deep tendon reflexes were brisk.

Given the clinical presentation, I suspected a progressive myoclonic epilepsy (PME), and Unverricht-Lundborg disease (ULD) was a leading consideration due to the age of onset and symptomatology. To confirm the diagnosis, I ordered a comprehensive set of diagnostic tests. The first step was to conduct an electroencephalogram (EEG) to evaluate the electrical activity in his brain. The EEG showed generalized spike-and-wave discharges, particularly during periods of myoclonic jerks and photic stimulation, consistent with a diagnosis of PME.

Next, I arranged for genetic testing to confirm the diagnosis of ULD. ULD is an autosomal recessive disorder caused by mutations in the CSTB gene, which encodes cystatin B, a protein involved in protease inhibition. The genetic test revealed homozygous mutations in the CSTB gene, confirming the diagnosis of Unverricht-Lundborg disease.

Once the diagnosis was established, I formulated a comprehensive treatment plan to manage the patient's symptoms and improve his quality of life. The primary goal of treatment in ULD is to control the myoclonic jerks and other seizure types, as well as to manage the ataxia and other neurological symptoms. I initiated the patient on valproic acid, which is the first-line treatment for myoclonic seizures in ULD. Valproic acid increases the availability of gamma-aminobutyric acid (GABA) in the brain, which helps to reduce neuronal excitability and suppress myoclonic jerks. The starting dose was 15 mg/kg/day, gradually titrated up to 60 mg/kg/day based on the patient's response and tolerability.

In addition to valproic acid, I prescribed clonazepam as an adjunctive therapy. Clonazepam is a benzodiazepine that enhances GABAergic transmission, providing additional control of myoclonic jerks. The initial dose was 0.5 mg/day, divided into two doses, and titrated up to 1.5 mg/day. I also advised the patient on the potential side effects of these medications, including drowsiness, dizziness, and gastrointestinal disturbances, and scheduled regular follow-up visits to monitor his response to treatment and adjust dosages as necessary.

To address the ataxia and coordination difficulties, I referred the patient to a physical therapist specializing in neurological disorders. The physical therapy regimen included exercises to improve balance, coordination, and strength, with the goal of enhancing his functional mobility and independence. Occupational therapy was also recommended to assist the patient in adapting daily activities and developing strategies to compensate for his motor impairments.

Given the progressive nature of ULD, it was crucial to monitor the patient's cognitive function regularly. While cognitive decline is not a primary feature of ULD, some patients may experience subtle cognitive changes over time. I conducted a baseline neuropsychological assessment to evaluate his cognitive status and planned for annual follow-ups to detect any changes early.

To provide comprehensive care, I also addressed the psychosocial aspects of the disease. The patient and his family were provided with information about ULD, including its genetic basis, prognosis, and available support resources. Genetic counseling was offered to the patient's family members to discuss the risk of recurrence in future generations and the availability of carrier testing.

Over the next few months, the patient's condition stabilized with the prescribed treatment regimen. The frequency and severity of his myoclonic jerks decreased significantly, allowing him to regain some control over his movements. His ataxia improved with physical therapy, and he reported fewer falls and increased confidence in performing daily activities. Despite these improvements, he continued to experience some degree of motor impairment and required ongoing support and adjustments to his treatment plan.

Unfortunately, as with many cases of ULD, the patient's condition began to deteriorate over time. After two years of relatively stable health, he started experiencing breakthrough myoclonic seizures despite optimal medical therapy. I adjusted his medication regimen, adding levetiracetam as an adjunctive treatment. Levetiracetam is an antiepileptic drug that modulates synaptic neurotransmitter release, providing an additional mechanism to control seizures. The starting dose was 500 mg twice daily, titrated up to 1500 mg twice daily.

Despite these efforts, the patient's neurological decline continued. He developed generalized tonic-clonic seizures, which became increasingly frequent and difficult to control. The addition of levetiracetam provided some relief, but the seizures persisted. His ataxia worsened, and he became wheelchair-bound. Cognitive assessments revealed a gradual decline in executive function and memory, although he remained oriented and communicative.

Given the refractory nature of his seizures and the progression of his neurological symptoms, I explored additional treatment options. One potential therapy for refractory myoclonic seizures is the ketogenic diet, a high-fat, low-carbohydrate diet that has been shown to reduce seizure frequency in some patients with epilepsy. I referred the patient to a dietitian experienced in managing ketogenic diets for epilepsy, and the diet was initiated under close medical supervision.

The ketogenic diet provided moderate seizure control, reducing the frequency of his tonic-clonic seizures and myoclonic jerks. However, the patient continued to experience significant disability due to his ataxia and cognitive decline. Over the next year, his condition remained relatively stable, but he required increasing assistance with daily activities and had frequent hospitalizations for seizure management and complications such as aspiration pneumonia.

Ultimately, the patient's condition continued to worsen despite all medical interventions. He developed status epilepticus, a life-threatening condition characterized by continuous or rapidly recurring seizures without recovery of consciousness between episodes. Despite aggressive treatment with intravenous antiepileptic drugs, including midazolam and propofol, his seizures could not be controlled.

The patient was admitted to the intensive care unit, where he was placed on continuous EEG monitoring and received high-dose antiepileptic medications. Despite these measures, he remained in status epilepticus, and his neurological function continued to deteriorate. After several weeks in the ICU, it became clear that his prognosis was poor, with little chance of recovery.

In consultation with the patient's family, a decision was made to withdraw aggressive treatment and provide palliative care to ensure his comfort. The focus shifted to managing his symptoms and providing emotional support to his family during this difficult time. The patient passed away peacefully a few days later, surrounded by his loved ones.

Despite our best efforts to manage his symptoms and improve his quality of life, the progressive and refractory nature of his seizures ultimately led to his decline and death. This case underscored the need for continued research into more effective therapies for ULD and other progressive myoclonic epilepsies, as well as the importance of providing comprehensive and compassionate care to patients and their families facing these devastating diseases.

❧ 17 ❧

TULAREMIA

When the patient first arrived at the clinic, their presentation was not immediately alarming, though it was certainly curious. The patient was a middle-aged individual, presenting with symptoms that initially seemed indicative of a common flu: fever, chills, and a general sense of malaise. However, upon closer examination, it became clear that this was no ordinary case of influenza.

The patient reported having been in the woods a few days prior, engaging in outdoor activities such as hiking and hunting. This detail, while seemingly mundane, proved crucial in the eventual diagnosis. The patient also mentioned having handled a rabbit carcass without gloves, which raised my suspicion further.

On physical examination, the patient exhibited a high fever of 104°F (40°C) and a markedly swollen and tender lymph node in the axillary region. The skin overlying the lymph node was erythematous but not fluctuating. The patient also had an ulcerative lesion on their hand, which they attributed to a minor cut sustained while handling the rabbit.

Given the combination of high fever, lymphadenopathy, and a recent history of contact with potentially infected animals, I considered several differential diagnoses. However, tularemia quickly rose to the top of the list. Tularemia, also known as rabbit fever, is caused by the bacterium Francisella tularensis, a highly infectious pathogen that can be transmitted through various means, including insect bites, handling of infected animals, ingestion of contaminated water, and inhalation of aerosols.

To confirm the diagnosis, I ordered several laboratory tests. A blood sample was sent for serology to detect antibodies against Francisella tularensis. Additionally, a sample from the ulcerative lesion was collected for culture and PCR testing. Given the high infectivity of the organism, all samples were handled with extreme caution, and appropriate biosafety protocols were followed to prevent laboratory-acquired infections.

While awaiting the laboratory results, I initiated empirical antibiotic therapy. Given the patient's presentation and my strong suspicion of tularemia, I started treatment with streptomycin, the antibiotic of choice for this infection. Streptomycin, an aminoglycoside antibiotic, is highly effective against Francisella tularensis and is typically administered intramuscularly. The dosage for adults is 1 gram twice daily for 10 days.

In addition to antibiotic therapy, I provided supportive care to manage the patient's symptoms. Antipyretics were administered to reduce the fever, and the patient was encouraged to stay well-hydrated. The swollen lymph node was monitored closely, though it did not appear to require surgical intervention at this stage.

The serological tests confirmed the diagnosis of tularemia. The patient had a significant rise in antibody titers against Francisella tularensis, consistent with an acute infection. The culture of the ulcerative lesion also grew Francisella tularensis, further confirming the diagnosis. Given the definitive laboratory confirmation, the treatment plan with streptomycin was continued.

Over the next few days, the patient began to show signs of improvement. The fever gradually subsided, and the tenderness and swelling of the lymph node decreased. The ulcerative lesion on the hand started to heal, with the edges becoming less erythematous and more defined.

Despite the positive response to treatment, tularemia can have a protracted course, and complications are not uncommon. I closely monitored the patient for any signs of potential complications, such as pneumonia, meningitis, or disseminated infection. Regular follow-up visits were scheduled to assess the patient's progress and ensure the infection was fully resolved.

Throughout the course of treatment, I emphasized the importance of completing the full 10-day course of antibiotics, even if symptoms resolved sooner. Incomplete treatment can lead to relapse or the development of antibiotic-resistant strains of Francisella tularensis. The patient adhered well to the treatment regimen, and no adverse effects from the streptomycin were observed.

In addition to the medical management, I provided the patient with education on preventing future infections. Given their history of outdoor activities and handling of wildlife, it was important to discuss measures such as wearing gloves when handling animals, using insect repellent to prevent tick bites, and ensuring proper cooking of game meat. Tularemia is a zoonotic disease, and understanding the modes of transmission is crucial in preventing recurrence.

At the end of the 10-day treatment course, the patient was reevaluated. They had made a remarkable recovery, with no residual symptoms. The fever had completely resolved, the lymphadenopathy had subsided, and the ulcerative lesion was healing well. Follow-up serological testing showed a decrease in antibody titers, indicating a resolving infection.

While the patient had a favorable outcome, tularemia can be a severe and potentially life-threatening illness if not promptly diagnosed and treated. The clinical presentation can vary widely, ranging from mild flu-like symptoms to severe systemic disease. Early recognition and appropriate antibiotic therapy are key to successful management.

Reflecting on this case, it reinforced the importance of taking a thorough history and considering zoonotic diseases in patients with relevant exposure histories. Tularemia, though rare, should be part of the differential diagnosis in patients presenting with fever, lymphadenopathy, and a history of contact with wildlife or outdoor activities.

This patient's case of tularemia was successfully diagnosed and treated with streptomycin, resulting in complete recovery.

A s a hematologist, my practice involved a variety of blood disorders, but a particular case of Thalassemia Major, also known as Cooley's Anemia, left a significant mark on my career. The patient, a young adult of Mediterranean descent, presented with severe anemia, jaundice, and noticeable skeletal deformities, particularly in the facial bones, which is often a telltale sign of this hereditary condition.

The patient had a history of persistent fatigue, pallor, and episodes of jaundice. Upon physical examination, the patient exhibited marked pallor, hepatosplenomegaly, and a distinctive frontal bossing and maxillary hyperplasia due to bone marrow expansion. The clinical suspicion of Thalassemia was strong, but confirmation required a thorough laboratory workup.

A complete blood count (CBC) revealed profound

microcytic hypochromic anemia with a hemoglobin level of 6.2 g/dL, a mean corpuscular volume (MCV) of 58 fL, and a mean corpuscular hemoglobin (MCH) of 19 pg. The reticulocyte count was elevated at 6%, indicating a compensatory increase in erythropoiesis. Peripheral blood smear showed anisopoikilocytosis, target cells, and nucleated red blood cells, which are characteristic of Thalassemia.

To confirm the diagnosis, hemoglobin electrophoresis was performed. The results showed markedly reduced levels of hemoglobin A (HbA), increased levels of hemoglobin F (HbF), and the presence of hemoglobin A2 (HbA2). These findings were indicative of β-Thalassemia Major. Genetic testing further confirmed the diagnosis, revealing mutations in both alleles of the HBB gene.

Given the severity of the condition, the patient required an aggressive and multidisciplinary approach. The cornerstone of managing Thalassemia Major involves regular blood transfusions, iron chelation therapy, and supportive measures to manage complications. Our initial treatment plan was structured as follows:

- Regular Blood Transfusions: The patient was started on a chronic transfusion regimen to maintain a pre-transfusion hemoglobin level above 9-10 g/dL. This aimed to suppress ineffective erythropoiesis and minimize bone marrow expansion. Transfusions were scheduled every three to four weeks, with careful monitoring for transfusion reactions and alloimmunization.

- Iron Chelation Therapy: Chronic transfusions inevitably lead to iron overload, which can cause significant damage to vital organs, particularly the liver, heart, and endocrine glands. The patient was started on iron chelation therapy with deferoxamine, administered subcutaneously via a portable pump over 8-12 hours daily. Regular monitoring of serum ferritin levels and liver iron concentration via MRI was planned to assess and adjust the chelation regimen.

- Splenectomy Consideration: Given the significant splenomegaly and hypersplenism, which contributed to increased red cell destruction and transfusion requirements, splenectomy was considered. However, due to the associated risks, including increased susceptibility to infections, this option was deferred and closely monitored.

- Folic Acid Supplementation: To support erythropoiesis, the patient was prescribed folic acid supplements. Folic acid is crucial in DNA synthesis and red blood cell production, and its supplementation is a standard adjunct in managing Thalassemia.

- Endocrine and Cardiac Monitoring: Regular assessments of endocrine function (including thyroid, glucose metabolism, and growth parameters) and cardiac evaluations were integral parts of the management plan. This involved periodic echocardiograms and endocrine function tests to detect and address complications early.
- Bone Marrow Transplant (BMT) Evaluation: The only curative treatment for Thalassemia Major is allogeneic hematopoietic stem cell transplantation. The patient was evaluated for suitability for a bone marrow transplant, including HLA typing and a search for a compatible donor among family members and the international donor registry. Given the complexities and risks associated with BMT, a thorough discussion with the patient and their family was conducted to weigh the benefits and potential complications.

Over the following months, the patient adhered to the transfusion schedule and iron chelation therapy. Regular monitoring showed effective maintenance of target hemoglobin levels and a gradual decrease in serum ferritin levels, indicating successful management of iron overload. However, the journey was not without challenges.

The patient experienced several transfusion reactions, managed with pre-medications and slow transfusion rates. Despite these precautions, alloimmunization occurred, necessitating more stringent cross-matching procedures and occasional use of immunosuppressive therapy.

A significant complication arose in the form of iron-induced cardiomyopathy, detected during a routine echocardiogram, which showed reduced ejection fraction. This led to the initiation of combination iron chelation therapy with the addition of deferasirox to intensify iron removal. Cardiac medications, including ACE inhibitors and beta-blockers, were also introduced to manage heart failure symptoms.

Endocrine complications were another hurdle. The patient developed hypothyroidism and diabetes mellitus, likely due to iron deposition in the thyroid and pancreatic islets. Levothyroxine and insulin therapy were started, with regular follow-up to titrate doses and monitor glucose control.

Despite these interventions, the patient's quality of life was significantly impacted by the chronic disease and its complications. The option of bone marrow transplantation remained a potential cure, but a suitable donor had not yet been identified.

Thalassemia Major is a lifelong condition requiring meticulous management. In this case, despite rigorous adherence to treatment protocols, the patient faced numerous complications that underscored the relentless nature of the disease. The iron chelation therapy, while reducing iron overload, brought its own set of challenges, including compliance issues due to the demanding administration schedule and side effects.

Regular follow-ups revealed a gradual stabilization of the patient's condition. However, the specter of further complications, such as progressive heart disease, liver cirrhosis, and endocrine dysfunction, loomed large. The patient's resilience and determination to adhere to the treatment regimen were commendable, but the relentless progression of the disease underscored the urgent need for a definitive cure.

The management of Thalassemia Major is a complex interplay of chronic transfusions, iron chelation, and vigilant monitoring for complications. Despite the aggressive treatment, the patient's condition remained precarious, and the hope for a bone marrow transplant as a potential cure was a constant undercurrent in the ongoing battle against the disease.

❧ 19 ❧

LOWE SYNDROME

As a pediatrician specializing in rare genetic disorders, I encountered a particularly challenging case of Lowe syndrome. This disorder, also known as oculocerebrorenal syndrome, is a rare condition affecting the eyes, brain, and kidneys, caused by mutations in the OCRL gene. The patient was a five-month-old male who presented with significant developmental delays, poor muscle tone, and distinct ocular abnormalities. The family history revealed no known genetic disorders, which indicated a de novo mutation.

Upon initial examination, the patient exhibited nystagmus, a condition where the eyes make repetitive, uncontrolled movements, reducing vision and depth perception. His ocular lens showed congenital cataracts, which are hallmark signs of Lowe syndrome. Further ophthalmologic evaluation confirmed bilateral dense cataracts. The patient also had microphthalmia, indicating smaller than normal eyes, a common characteristic in Lowe syndrome patients.

The neurological assessment revealed hypotonia, a state of low muscle tone, particularly evident in the axial muscles, affecting the patient's ability to maintain head control and sit without support. The patient's developmental milestones were significantly delayed; he had not yet begun to roll over, babble, or grasp objects, which are typical activities for his age group. Reflex testing showed decreased deep tendon reflexes, another sign consistent with hypotonia.

Given the constellation of symptoms, I ordered a series of diagnostic tests. A comprehensive metabolic panel was conducted to assess the kidney function, as Lowe syndrome often involves renal tubular dysfunction. The results showed elevated levels of amino acids, glucose, bicarbonate, and phosphate in the urine, indicative of Fanconi syndrome, which is frequently associated with Lowe syndrome. Blood tests revealed normal serum electrolytes but a slight acidosis, further supporting the diagnosis of renal tubular dysfunction.

Genetic testing was the definitive step in confirming Lowe syndrome. A blood sample was sent for sequencing of the OCRL gene. The results came back positive for a mutation in exon 8 of the OCRL gene, confirming the diagnosis of Lowe syndrome.

The treatment plan for Lowe syndrome is multidisciplinary, involving ophthalmologic, nephrologic, neurologic, and supportive care. The first step was addressing the congenital cataracts to prevent further visual impairment. An ophthalmologist performed bilateral cataract extraction surgery. Post-surgical care included wearing protective eye patches and administering antibiotic and anti-inflammatory eye drops to prevent infection and inflammation.

The renal complications required a comprehensive approach to manage Fanconi syndrome. The patient was started on oral supplements to correct the electrolyte imbalances, including sodium bicarbonate to manage acidosis, potassium chloride for hypokalemia, and phosphate supplements for hypophosphatemia. Additionally, vitamin D and calcium supplements were prescribed to prevent bone demineralization, a common consequence of renal tubular acidosis.

Managing hypotonia involved a rigorous physical and occupational therapy regimen. Physical therapy sessions focused on strengthening the axial muscles, improving head control, and enhancing gross motor skills. Occupational therapy aimed to develop fine motor skills and improve the patient's ability to perform daily activities. The patient's caregivers were trained to perform specific exercises at home to reinforce the therapy sessions.

Neurologically, the patient was monitored for signs of developmental delay and intellectual disability. A pediatric neurologist was consulted to provide ongoing assessment and intervention. Regular developmental assessments were scheduled to monitor progress and adjust the therapeutic interventions as needed.

Nutrition played a crucial role in the patient's overall health. Due to the increased risk of growth retardation and malnutrition in children with Lowe syndrome, a dietitian was involved to ensure adequate caloric and nutritional intake. A high-calorie diet was recommended, with frequent small meals rich in proteins and essential nutrients. In cases where oral intake was insufficient, a gastrostomy tube might be considered, but fortunately, the patient maintained adequate oral intake.

Regular follow-up appointments were crucial in managing this complex condition. The patient was scheduled for monthly visits to monitor growth parameters, kidney function, and developmental milestones. Every three months, he underwent a comprehensive metabolic panel to assess the efficacy of the renal treatment and adjust supplements as needed. Ophthalmologic evaluations were also conducted every three months to monitor for potential complications such as glaucoma, which is a risk following cataract surgery in patients with Lowe syndrome.

Despite the intensive medical and supportive care, the prognosis for Lowe syndrome remains guarded. The progressive nature of the disorder, particularly the renal and neurological aspects, poses significant challenges. The patient continued to experience developmental delays, though some progress was noted with the dedicated therapeutic interventions. His muscle tone improved marginally, allowing for better head control and the ability to sit with support.

At the age of three, the patient developed nephrocalcinosis, a condition characterized by calcium deposits in the kidneys. This was detected during routine ultrasound imaging. The condition was managed by adjusting his dietary intake and increasing his hydration to prevent kidney stones and further renal damage. Unfortunately, this added another layer of complexity to his already challenging condition.

By age four, the patient's renal function began to decline, as evidenced by rising serum creatinine levels and worsening electrolyte imbalances despite aggressive management. The family was counseled about the progressive nature of renal disease in Lowe syndrome and the potential need for renal replacement therapy in the future.

As the patient reached five years of age, his cognitive and physical development remained significantly delayed. He achieved limited verbal communication and required assistance for most daily activities. The physical therapy sessions continued to focus on maintaining muscle tone and preventing contractures, while occupational therapy aimed at maximizing his functional abilities within the scope of his condition.

Tragically, at the age of six, the patient developed

end-stage renal disease (ESRD), a known severe complication of Lowe syndrome. Despite all efforts to manage his condition conservatively, it was clear that he would need dialysis to sustain life. Hemodialysis was initiated, but the procedure posed significant challenges given his young age and small body size.

The patient's overall condition continued to deteriorate. The combination of ESRD, severe developmental delays, and complications from dialysis led to frequent hospitalizations. His immune system was compromised, making him susceptible to infections, which further complicated his treatment.

Ultimately, the patient succumbed to his condition at the age of seven, passing away due to complications from a severe systemic infection that his weakened body could not withstand.

The experience reaffirmed the importance of early diagnosis, a multidisciplinary approach to care, and the need for ongoing research to develop better treatments for rare genetic disorders like Lowe syndrome. It also underscored the resilience and dedication of the families who care for children with such challenging conditions, as they navigate the complexities of managing a rare and devastating illness.

The patient came to my office with a primary complaint of multiple skin lesions that had been present since childhood but had significantly increased in number and size over the past few years. A physical examination revealed numerous café-au-lait spots, which are flat, pigmented birthmarks, spread across the patient's body. Additionally, there were several neurofibromas, benign nerve sheath tumors, that varied in size and were particularly noticeable on the trunk and extremities.

Neurofibromatosis type 1 (NF1), also known as von Recklinghausen's disease, is an autosomal dominant genetic disorder. The hallmark of NF1 is the development of multiple benign tumors of the nerves and skin (neurofibromas) and areas of abnormal skin pigmentation (café-au-lait spots). The NF1 gene, located on chromosome 17, encodes a protein called neurofibromin, which acts as a tumor suppressor. Mutations in this gene lead to a lack of functional neurofibromin, resulting in the formation of tumors along nerves in the skin, brain, and other parts of the body.

The diagnosis of NF1 is primarily clinical, based on criteria established by the National Institutes of Health (NIH). For a diagnosis of NF1, at least two of the following criteria must be met:

1. Six or more café-au-lait macules larger than 5 mm in prepubertal individuals and larger than 15 mm in postpubertal individuals.
2. Two or more neurofibromas of any type or one plexiform neurofibroma.
3. Freckling in the axillary or inguinal regions.
4. Optic glioma.
5. Two or more Lisch nodules (iris hamartomas).
6. A distinctive osseous lesion such as sphenoid dysplasia or thinning of long bone cortex with or without pseudarthrosis.
7. A first-degree relative (parent, sibling, or offspring) with NF1 based on the above criteria.

The patient exhibited six café-au-lait spots larger than 15 mm and multiple neurofibromas, meeting the NIH criteria for NF1. Additional diagnostic tests were conducted to assess the extent of the disease. A thorough ophthalmological examination revealed Lisch nodules, which are benign growths on the iris. MRI of the brain and spinal cord was performed to check for the presence of optic gliomas or other central nervous system abnormalities, common in NF1 patients. Fortunately, no optic gliomas were detected, but the MRI did show a small lesion in the left parietal lobe, suggesting a possible low-grade glioma.

The patient also underwent a skeletal survey to identify any bony abnormalities. The X-rays showed mild scoliosis but no significant osseous lesions. Genetic testing was offered to confirm the diagnosis, but the patient declined, given the clear clinical picture and the financial constraints involved.

Management of NF1 is primarily focused on symptomatic relief and monitoring for complications. Given the presence of multiple neurofibromas and their potential for causing pain, disfigurement, or functional impairment, a multidisciplinary approach was recommended.

The patient was referred to a dermatologist for management of the skin lesions. Surgical removal of the larger neurofibromas was considered to alleviate discomfort and reduce the risk of malignant transformation, although the risk is generally low. The patient was advised that surgery could be repeated as needed due to the likelihood of new neurofibroma development. Pain management was an important aspect, as neurofibromas can sometimes compress nerves, causing significant discomfort. Gabapentin was prescribed for neuropathic pain, starting at a low dose of 300 mg daily and gradually increased to 900 mg daily, depending on the patient's response and tolerance.

Regular follow-up with an ophthalmologist was necessary to monitor for the development of optic gliomas and other eye-related complications. Annual eye exams were scheduled to detect any changes early. The patient was also advised to have periodic MRIs of the brain and spine to monitor the existing glioma and to screen for any new central nervous system tumors. Given the small size and stable appearance of the glioma, a watch-and-wait approach was adopted, with imaging every six months.

The patient was educated about the importance of regular skin checks to monitor for changes in existing neurofibromas and the appearance of new lesions. Instructions were given on how to self-examine and what signs to look out for, such as rapid growth, color change, or ulceration, which could indicate malignant transformation.

A referral to a genetic counselor was made to discuss the implications of NF1 for the patient's family. As NF1 is an autosomal dominant condition, each offspring has a 50% chance of inheriting the disorder. The genetic counselor could provide information on family planning options, including prenatal testing and preimplantation genetic diagnosis.

Given the patient's mild scoliosis, regular follow-up with an orthopedic specialist was recommended to monitor for progression. Physical therapy was suggested to maintain strength and flexibility, and to manage any pain associated with the scoliosis. The patient was also encouraged to maintain a healthy lifestyle, including regular exercise, a balanced diet, and avoidance of smoking, which can exacerbate complications of NF1.

Over the next few years, the patient adhered to the management plan with regular follow-ups and imaging studies. The neurofibromas remained mostly stable in size, although a few new lesions did appear, which were managed surgically. The patient reported good pain control with gabapentin, and no significant side effects were noted. The small glioma in the left parietal lobe showed no signs of growth or malignant transformation on serial MRIs, and the patient remained asymptomatic with regard to neurological function.

Psychological support was also an important aspect of care, as chronic conditions like NF1 can have a significant impact on mental health. The patient was referred to a psychologist for counseling to help cope with the emotional burden of living with a chronic, potentially disfiguring condition. The patient found these sessions beneficial and reported improved mood and coping strategies.

Unfortunately, several years into the follow-up, the patient began to experience worsening headaches and vision changes. An urgent MRI revealed that the previously stable glioma had started to grow, with features suggestive of a higher-grade malignancy. A biopsy confirmed the diagnosis of a malignant peripheral nerve sheath tumor (MPNST), a known but rare complication of NF1.

The patient was referred to an oncologist for further management. A treatment plan was developed, which included surgery to remove as much of the tumor as possible, followed by radiation therapy and chemotherapy. The surgical team was able to achieve a near-total resection of the tumor, but the aggressive nature of MPNST meant that adjunctive therapy was necessary.

Radiation therapy was administered to the tumor bed to reduce the risk of recurrence. Chemotherapy was initiated with a regimen commonly used for MPNST, including doxorubicin and ifosfamide. The patient tolerated the initial cycles of chemotherapy well, with manageable side effects such as fatigue, nausea, and mild neuropathy.

Despite aggressive treatment, follow-up imaging revealed metastasis to the lungs, a common site for MPNST spread. Palliative care was introduced to manage symptoms and improve quality of life. Pain management became a primary focus, with a combination of opioids and adjuvant medications to control pain effectively.

The patient's condition continued to decline over the

next few months. The metastases in the lungs progressed, leading to respiratory compromise. Despite all efforts, the patient succumbed to the disease approximately six months after the diagnosis of MPNST.

Neurofibromatosis type 1 is a complex disorder with a wide range of manifestations and potential complications. In this case, despite careful monitoring and a comprehensive treatment plan, the patient developed a severe complication that ultimately proved fatal.

HANTAVIRUS PULMONARY SYNDROME

When the patient first came to my attention, they were already in a state of significant respiratory distress. As a rural physician, I had seen my fair share of respiratory illnesses, but this one immediately struck me as unusual. The patient, a middle-aged individual, presented with a sudden onset of fever, muscle aches, and fatigue, symptoms that could easily be mistaken for influenza. However, it was the rapid progression to severe shortness of breath that raised my suspicion.

Upon examination, the patient was febrile, with a temperature of 102.5°F, and had tachypnea with a respiratory rate of 30 breaths per minute. Their blood pressure was low at 90/60 mmHg, and they had a heart rate of 110 beats per minute, indicating tachycardia. Auscultation of the lungs revealed crackles and decreased breath sounds bilaterally, suggestive of pulmonary edema. Given the acute onset and severity of symptoms, I immediately considered a differential diagnosis that included acute respiratory distress syndrome (ARDS), bacterial or viral pneumonia, and other severe respiratory infections.

A detailed history from the patient revealed that they lived in a rural area and had been cleaning out a rodent-infested barn a few weeks prior to the onset of symptoms. This detail was crucial, as it pointed towards a possible hantavirus infection, a rare but serious respiratory disease transmitted by rodents.

I ordered a series of diagnostic tests, including a complete blood count (CBC), blood cultures, chest X-ray, and serologic testing for hantavirus. The CBC showed thrombocytopenia with a platelet count of 100,000/µL, hemoconcentration with a hematocrit of 55%, and leukocytosis with a white blood cell count of 15,000/µL. These findings were consistent with hantavirus pulmonary syndrome (HPS), which is characterized by an increase in hematocrit and a decrease in platelets due to vascular permeability and fluid leakage into the lungs.

The chest X-ray revealed bilateral interstitial infiltrates and evidence of pulmonary edema, further supporting the diagnosis of HPS. Blood cultures were negative, ruling out bacterial infection as a primary cause. The definitive diagnosis was confirmed by positive serologic tests for hantavirus-specific IgM and IgG antibodies.

With the diagnosis established, the treatment plan focused on supportive care, as there is no specific antiviral therapy for HPS. The patient was admitted to the intensive care unit (ICU) for close monitoring and aggressive supportive treatment. This included supplemental oxygen to maintain adequate oxygenation, intravenous fluids to support blood pressure and prevent shock, and careful monitoring of fluid balance to avoid exacerbating the pulmonary edema.

Given the severity of the patient's respiratory distress, I consulted with the critical care team and decided to initiate mechanical ventilation. Intubation was performed to secure the airway, and the patient was placed on a ventilator with settings optimized to reduce lung injury. We used a low tidal volume ventilation strategy to minimize barotrauma and volutrauma, which are critical in managing ARDS and conditions like HPS.

Fluid management was a delicate balance. While it was essential to maintain adequate intravascular volume to support blood pressure, excessive fluid administration could worsen pulmonary edema. We monitored the patient's central venous pressure and urine output closely, adjusting intravenous fluid administration accordingly. A central venous catheter was placed for accurate hemodynamic monitoring and to administer vasoactive medications if needed.

To address potential complications, we started prophylactic antibiotics to prevent secondary bacterial infections, which are common in patients with severe respiratory illnesses. We also administered low-dose corticosteroids to mitigate the inflammatory response, although their benefit in HPS is not well established and remains controversial.

Over the next several days, the patient remained critically ill but stable on mechanical ventilation. We performed daily assessments, including arterial blood gases, chest X-rays, and regular monitoring of electrolytes, renal function, and liver function. The patient's condition fluctuated, with periods of relative stability followed by episodes of increased respiratory distress and hypoxemia.

Despite our best efforts, the patient developed acute renal failure, a known complication of HPS due to the systemic capillary leak syndrome and reduced perfusion to the kidneys. Continuous renal replacement therapy (CRRT) was initiated to manage the renal failure and maintain fluid balance. CRRT allowed for gentle fluid removal and helped control the electrolyte imbalances that arose as a consequence of both the disease and the treatment.

We faced another challenge when the patient developed disseminated intravascular coagulation (DIC), a severe condition characterized by widespread activation of the coagulation cascade, leading to both thrombosis and bleeding. The patient's platelet count continued to drop, and they developed petechiae and ecchymoses. To manage DIC, we administered platelet transfusions, fresh frozen plasma, and cryoprecipitate as needed, while closely monitoring coagulation parameters and adjusting treatment based on the clinical picture.

Throughout the course of the illness, we provided the patient with nutritional support via a nasogastric tube, ensuring they received adequate calories and protein to support healing and recovery. This was vital, as the metabolic demands of severe illness are high, and malnutrition could further complicate the clinical course.

After approximately two weeks of intensive care, the patient began to show signs of improvement. Their oxygenation stabilized, and we were able to gradually wean them off the ventilator. The renal function started to recover, and the need for CRRT decreased. With careful management of fluids and electrolytes, the patient's condition continued to stabilize.

Eventually, the patient was extubated and transitioned to high-flow nasal cannula oxygen therapy. Over the following days, their respiratory function improved significantly, allowing us to reduce and finally discontinue supplemental oxygen. The patient was transferred out of the ICU to a step-down unit for further recovery.

During their stay in the step-down unit, the patient continued to improve and was able to start ambulating with the assistance of physical therapy. We monitored their progress closely, ensuring that any residual effects of the illness were addressed, including potential psychological impacts such as post-traumatic stress disorder (PTSD) from the prolonged ICU stay.

By the time the patient was discharged from the hospital, they had made a remarkable recovery. Follow-up appointments were scheduled to monitor long-term recovery and to manage any lingering health issues. The patient was advised to avoid further exposure to rodent-infested areas and to take precautions to prevent future hantavirus infection.

While there is no specific antiviral treatment for hantavirus, meticulous management of respiratory and hemodynamic parameters, along with vigilant monitoring for complications, was crucial in ensuring the patient's survival.

The patient's journey through hantavirus pulmonary syndrome was fraught with challenges, from initial diagnosis to the management of severe complications. However, with careful and coordinated medical care, they were able to recover and eventually return to their normal life.

❧ 22 ❧
TOGAVIRIDAE INFECTION

T he patient came into the clinic with symptoms that had been escalating over the past few days. Initially, the patient experienced a mild fever and headache, but these symptoms had progressed to severe joint pain and a pronounced rash. The presentation of these symptoms, coupled with the patient's recent travel history to a region known for mosquito-borne illnesses, raised my suspicion of a Togaviridae infection. Togaviridae encompasses several significant viruses, including Chikungunya and Ross River virus, which are known to cause such clinical manifestations.

Upon initial examination, the patient exhibited a high-grade fever of 39.5°C (103.1°F), conjunctival injection, and lymphadenopathy. The rash was erythematous and maculopapular, spreading across the torso and extremities. Joint pain was predominantly in the wrists, knees, and ankles, and the patient described the pain as debilitating, significantly impairing mobility.

A detailed patient history revealed recent travel to Southeast Asia, where Chikungunya virus (CHIKV) is endemic. This information, combined with the clinical presentation, made CHIKV the primary suspect. Laboratory tests were promptly ordered, including complete blood count (CBC), liver function tests (LFTs), and a polymerase chain reaction (PCR) test specifically for Chikungunya virus.

The CBC revealed leukopenia with a white blood cell count of 3,000/mm^3, thrombocytopenia with a platelet count of 120,000/mm^3, and mild anemia with a hemoglobin level of 11.2 g/dL. LFTs indicated elevated liver enzymes, with alanine transaminase (ALT) at 80 U/L and aspartate transaminase (AST) at 95 U/L, suggestive of hepatic involvement. The PCR test confirmed the presence of Chikungunya virus RNA, solidifying the diagnosis of CHIKV infection.

The primary treatment goal for Chikungunya is symptomatic relief, as there are no antiviral medications specifically targeting the virus. The management plan included antipyretics to control fever and analgesics to alleviate joint pain. Paracetamol (acetaminophen) was prescribed at 500 mg every six hours as needed for fever and pain. Nonsteroidal anti-inflammatory drugs (NSAIDs) were initially considered for joint pain, but due to the patient's thrombocytopenia, they were contraindicated to avoid the risk of bleeding.

Hydration was emphasized to support renal function and maintain electrolyte balance, given the patient's fever and potential for dehydration. The patient was advised to consume at least two liters of fluids per day, including oral rehydration solutions to replenish electrolytes lost through perspiration.

Given the patient's significant joint pain and potential for long-term arthralgia, a short course of corticosteroids was considered. Prednisone was prescribed at 20 mg daily for five days, followed by a tapering dose over the next week. This decision was made to reduce inflammation and improve joint function, with careful monitoring for potential side effects such as hyperglycemia and immunosuppression.

Rest was strongly recommended to facilitate recovery. The patient was advised to avoid strenuous activities and to elevate the affected joints when possible to reduce swelling. Light, gentle movements were encouraged to maintain joint flexibility and prevent stiffness.

Throughout the course of treatment, the patient was monitored closely for signs of complications. Serial CBC and LFTs were performed every three days to track any changes in hematologic and hepatic parameters. Fortunately, the patient's liver enzyme levels stabilized and began to decline within a week, indicating a positive response to the supportive care provided.

The patient's fever subsided within four days of initiating treatment, and the intensity of the rash decreased significantly. Joint pain, however, remained a persistent issue. The corticosteroid therapy provided some relief, but the patient continued to experience moderate discomfort, particularly in the mornings.

Physical therapy was introduced to assist with joint mobility and pain management. Gentle range-of-motion exercises were tailored to the patient's capabilities, focusing on reducing stiffness and improving function. The patient was instructed to perform these exercises twice daily and to use hot and cold compresses alternately to manage pain and swelling.

After three weeks of comprehensive care, the patient's condition improved markedly. The rash had completely resolved, fever was no longer present, and joint pain had diminished to a manageable level, allowing the patient to resume most daily activities. A follow-up PCR test for Chikungunya virus RNA was negative, indicating viral clearance.

The patient was discharged with instructions for continued physical therapy and periodic follow-ups to monitor for any long-term sequelae. Chronic joint pain, a known complication of CHIKV infection, was discussed, and the patient was advised to report any resurgence of symptoms immediately.

In the months following discharge, the patient's recovery trajectory remained positive. Joint pain continued to improve with physical therapy, and no further complications were observed. By the six-month mark, the patient reported only occasional mild joint discomfort, primarily in the mornings, which was effectively managed with intermittent use of acetaminophen.

Although the patient experienced a challenging recovery period marked by significant joint pain, the outcome was ultimately favorable, with no long-term disabilities or severe complications.

In conclusion, the patient's successful recovery from Chikungunya virus infection was a testament to the efficacy of a well-coordinated medical approach. While the absence of targeted antiviral therapy posed challenges, the principles of symptomatic relief, supportive care, and patient education facilitated a positive outcome. This experience reinforced my understanding of the complexities of managing viral infections and the necessity of a holistic, patient-centered approach in clinical practice.

WALDENSTROM MACROGLOBULINEMIA

As a hematologist, I encountered a case of Waldenstrom macroglobulinemia (WM) that stands out in my career due to its complexity and the challenges it presented. The patient was a 67-year-old male who was referred to my clinic for evaluation of persistent fatigue, weight loss, and night sweats. Upon reviewing his medical history, it was noted that he had been experiencing these symptoms for the past six months. Additionally, he had developed a progressive increase in abdominal girth and occasional episodes of epistaxis (nosebleeds).

During the initial physical examination, the patient appeared pale and had noticeable splenomegaly, with the spleen palpable approximately 5 cm below the left costal margin. There were no signs of lymphadenopathy. His vital signs were stable, but his overall appearance suggested a chronic illness. Given the constellation of symptoms and physical findings, I suspected an underlying hematologic disorder and proceeded with a comprehensive workup.

Initial laboratory tests revealed a normocytic, normochromic anemia with a hemoglobin level of 9.2 g/dL, a white blood cell count of 4.5 x 10^9/L, and a platelet count of 95 x 10^9/L. The erythrocyte sedimentation rate (ESR) was markedly elevated at 100 mm/hr, and the lactate dehydrogenase (LDH) level was also elevated. Serum protein electrophoresis (SPEP) demonstrated a monoclonal spike in the gamma region, suggestive of a monoclonal gammopathy. Further immunofixation electrophoresis confirmed the presence of an IgM monoclonal protein.

To further characterize the extent of the disease, I ordered a bone marrow biopsy and aspiration. The bone marrow biopsy showed hypercellularity with an interstitial infiltrate of small lymphoplasmacytic cells. The aspirate revealed the presence of lymphoplasmacytic lymphoma cells, and flow cytometry confirmed the clonal B-cell population expressing CD19, CD20, CD22, and surface immunoglobulin light chains. The MYD88 L265P mutation, commonly associated with WM, was also detected. These findings confirmed the diagnosis of Waldenstrom macroglobulinemia.

Given the diagnosis, the next step was to determine the staging and extent of disease involvement. Imaging studies, including a CT scan of the chest, abdomen, and pelvis, were performed. The CT scan revealed moderate hepatosplenomegaly but no significant lymphadenopathy. There were no lytic bone lesions or other extranodal involvements. Serum viscosity was measured due to the high IgM levels, and it was found to be elevated at 4.5 cP, raising concerns for hyperviscosity syndrome.

With the diagnosis established and the extent of disease involvement assessed, I formulated a treatment plan. The primary goals of treatment for WM are to reduce tumor burden, manage symptoms, and prevent complications such as hyperviscosity syndrome. Considering the patient's symptomatic hyperviscosity, immediate therapeutic intervention was necessary. Plasmapheresis was initiated to rapidly reduce the serum IgM levels and alleviate the symptoms related to hyperviscosity. The patient underwent two sessions of plasmapheresis, which resulted in significant improvement in his symptoms and a reduction in serum viscosity.

Following the plasmapheresis, I initiated systemic therapy to target the underlying disease. The standard first-line treatment for WM includes a combination of rituximab and chemotherapy. I opted for the DRC regimen, which consists of dexamethasone, rituximab, and cyclophosphamide. Dexamethasone was administered at a dose of 20 mg orally on days 1-4, rituximab at 375 mg/m^2 intravenously on day 1, and cyclophosphamide at

100 mg/m^2 orally on days 1-5, repeated every 21 days for six cycles.

Throughout the treatment course, the patient was monitored closely for any adverse effects and response to therapy. Common side effects of the DRC regimen include cytopenias, infections, and infusion-related reactions to rituximab. Prophylactic antimicrobial therapy, including acyclovir and trimethoprim-sulfamethoxazole, was prescribed to reduce the risk of infections. The patient tolerated the treatment well, with manageable side effects, primarily consisting of mild neutropenia and transient fatigue.

During the treatment, the patient's hemoglobin levels gradually improved, and his splenomegaly regressed. Serial serum protein electrophoresis and immunofixation showed a significant reduction in the IgM monoclonal protein levels. By the end of the six cycles of DRC, the patient achieved a partial response, with a more than 50% reduction in serum IgM levels and improvement in clinical symptoms.

Following the initial treatment, the patient entered a period of close surveillance. WM is a chronic, indolent disease with a relapsing-remitting course, and ongoing monitoring is essential. The patient was scheduled for regular follow-up visits every three months, which included physical examinations, complete blood counts, liver function tests, serum protein electrophoresis, and periodic imaging studies.

Approximately two years after the initial diagnosis, the patient experienced a relapse, with recurrent fatigue, anemia, and an increase in serum IgM levels. At this point, I decided to initiate a second-line therapy with a combination of bendamustine and rituximab. Bendamustine was administered at a dose of 90 mg/m^2 intravenously on days 1 and 2, and rituximab at 375 mg/m^2 intravenously on day 1, repeated every 28 days for six cycles.

The patient responded well to the second-line therapy, achieving another partial response with significant improvement in symptoms and a reduction in IgM levels. Despite the chronic nature of WM, the patient managed to maintain a good quality of life with periodic treatment and supportive care.

As the disease progressed over the years, the patient eventually developed refractory disease, which did not respond adequately to standard therapies. At this stage, the treatment strategy shifted towards palliative care to manage symptoms and improve quality of life. The patient received supportive care, including blood transfusions for anemia, analgesics for bone pain, and measures to manage infections and other complications.

Ultimately, after a prolonged and challenging battle with WM, the patient succumbed to the disease approximately five years after the initial diagnosis. The final stages were marked by significant cytopenias, recurrent infections, and organ dysfunction. Despite the advanced therapies available, the indolent yet relentless nature of WM ultimately led to the patient's demise.

While advances in therapy have improved outcomes for many patients with WM, it remains an incurable disease with a chronic course. The goal of treatment is to achieve symptom control, prolong survival, and maintain quality of life, even as we continue to search for more effective and definitive therapies.

❧ 24 ❧

AMBRAS SYNDROME

The patient was a 22-year-old male who presented to my clinic with an unusual and rare condition. He was referred to me by a general practitioner who had noticed excessive hair growth over most of his body, a condition known medically as hypertrichosis. This extreme and pervasive hair growth, which covered the patient's face, arms, back, and legs, was a significant concern, not only because of the physical appearance but also due to potential underlying genetic or systemic causes.

Upon initial examination, I observed that the patient's hair growth was dense and lanugo-like, similar to the fine hair that covers a fetus and typically sheds before birth. The patient's face, in particular, was almost entirely covered with this fine hair, leaving only small patches of visible skin. His eyebrows and eyelashes were also excessively thick. Despite the striking presentation, the patient was otherwise healthy, with no complaints of systemic symptoms such as weight loss, fever, or fatigue.

I proceeded with a thorough medical history, querying about the onset of symptoms, any familial history of similar conditions, and any associated symptoms that might indicate a broader syndrome. The patient reported that the hair growth had been present since birth and had progressively worsened with age. There was no family history of hypertrichosis or any other genetic disorders. This suggested a congenital form of hypertrichosis, likely genetic in nature.

To confirm the diagnosis, I ordered a series of tests, including a full genetic workup, complete blood count (CBC), metabolic panel, and hormone levels to rule out endocrine causes such as thyroid dysfunction or androgen excess. The genetic analysis revealed a mutation in the TRPS1 gene, a known cause of Ambras syndrome, a rare form of congenital hypertrichosis. This syndrome is characterized by generalized hypertrichosis, facial dysmorphism, and dental anomalies. In the patient's case, the hypertrichosis was the most prominent feature, with only mild facial dysmorphism and no significant dental issues.

The diagnosis of Ambras syndrome was confirmed, and I discussed the nature of the condition with the patient, explaining that it was a lifelong genetic disorder with no cure. Treatment would focus on managing the symptoms and improving quality of life. Given the extensive hair growth, I proposed a multi-faceted treatment plan involving dermatology and genetic counseling.

For immediate management of the hypertrichosis, I recommended a combination of laser hair removal and topical treatments. Laser hair removal, although not permanent, could significantly reduce the hair density and improve cosmetic appearance. The patient was referred to a dermatologist specializing in laser treatments, and an initial series of sessions was scheduled to assess the response. Topical eflornithine cream, an inhibitor of ornithine decarboxylase, was prescribed to slow down the rate of hair growth. The patient was instructed to apply the cream twice daily to the affected areas of the face and neck.

Additionally, I referred the patient to a genetic counselor to provide support and education about the condition and its hereditary nature. This would also include discussions about family planning and the risks of passing the condition to future offspring.

The patient underwent the first series of laser hair removal treatments over the next several months. The sessions were moderately painful but tolerable, and the patient reported a noticeable reduction in hair density. The topical eflornithine cream also proved effective in slowing new hair growth, although it did not eliminate it entirely. The combination of these treatments significantly improved the patient's cosmetic appearance and reduced the social and psychological burden of the condition.

Regular follow-ups were scheduled to monitor the effectiveness of the treatment and to manage any side effects. The patient reported occasional skin irritation and redness from the laser treatments, which was managed with topical corticosteroids and moisturizers. There were no significant adverse effects from the eflornithine cream.

In the long term, the patient's condition remained stable with ongoing laser treatments every few months and continuous use of the eflornithine cream. Genetic counseling provided valuable support and coping strategies, helping the patient adjust to living with Ambras syndrome. While the treatments did not cure the condition, they significantly improved the patient's quality of life, allowing him to lead a more normal and socially active life.

Over the course of several years, the patient's management plan was adjusted based on the response to treatments and any new developments in the field of dermatology and genetics. Emerging treatments, such as advanced laser technologies and potential gene therapies, were considered and discussed with the patient as part of ongoing care.

The condition, being genetic and congenital, required lifelong management, but with appropriate treatment and support, the patient was able to lead a fulfilling life despite the challenges posed by the syndrome.

❧ 25 ❧

ADULT T-CELL LEUKEMIA/LYMPHOMA

The patient was a 47-year-old male who presented to our clinic with complaints of generalized fatigue, significant weight loss over the past three months, night sweats, and a persistent rash. His past medical history was unremarkable except for a minor bout of pneumonia a few years prior. Given his nonspecific symptoms and the presence of a rash, our initial differential diagnosis included a range of possibilities from infectious etiologies to autoimmune disorders and malignancies.

On physical examination, the patient appeared cachectic and pale. He had multiple enlarged lymph nodes in the cervical, axillary, and inguinal regions. The rash was erythematous and maculopapular, covering his trunk and extremities. There was no hepatosplenomegaly, but his abdomen was mildly distended.

Initial laboratory investigations showed a white blood cell count of 22,000/µL with an abnormal differential revealing atypical lymphocytes. Hemoglobin was 9.8 g/dL, and platelets were 145,000/µL. Liver function tests indicated mild transaminitis. LDH was significantly elevated at 620 IU/L, and serum calcium was elevated at 11.5 mg/dL. These findings prompted further investigation with imaging studies.

A contrast-enhanced CT scan of the chest, abdomen, and pelvis revealed widespread lymphadenopathy, notably in the mediastinal, retroperitoneal, and pelvic regions. Additionally, lytic lesions were seen in the spine and pelvic bones, suggesting possible bone involvement. Given the constellation of symptoms and findings, we proceeded with a lymph node biopsy to obtain a definitive diagnosis.

The histopathological examination of the lymph node biopsy revealed effacement of the nodal architecture by a diffuse infiltrate of atypical lymphocytes with irregular nuclear contours, consistent with a T-cell lineage. Immunohistochemistry showed these cells were positive for CD2, CD3, CD4, and CD25, and negative for CD7 and CD8. The proliferation index, measured by Ki-67 staining, was high at 70%. These findings were consistent with Adult T-cell leukemia/lymphoma (ATLL), particularly of the acute subtype, given the high white cell count, hypercalcemia, and aggressive clinical course.

A confirmatory test for HTLV-1 (Human T-cell lymphotropic virus type 1) was positive, establishing the viral etiology of the malignancy. ATLL is a rare and aggressive form of peripheral T-cell lymphoma caused by HTLV-1, characterized by a poor prognosis.

Given the aggressive nature of the disease, we formulated a comprehensive treatment plan. The treatment strategy for ATLL is multifaceted, involving combination chemotherapy, antiviral therapy, and supportive care.

We initiated the patient on the CHOP regimen, which includes Cyclophosphamide, Doxorubicin, Vincristine, and Prednisone. Cyclophosphamide was administered at 750 mg/m^2 IV on day 1, Doxorubicin at 50 mg/m^2 IV on day 1, Vincristine at 1.4 mg/m^2 (max 2 mg) IV on day 1, and Prednisone at 100 mg orally daily on days 1-5. This cycle was to be repeated every 21 days for six cycles.

In parallel with chemotherapy, we started the patient on antiviral therapy with Zidovudine (AZT) and Interferon-alpha, as studies have shown this combination can provide a survival benefit in patients with acute and lymphoma subtypes of ATLL. Zidovudine was given at a dose of 600 mg/day in divided doses, and Interferon-alpha was administered at 3 million units subcutaneously three times per week.

Supportive care measures included aggressive hydration and bisphosphonate therapy with Pamidronate to manage hypercalcemia, as well as prophylactic antibiotics to prevent opportunistic infections due to immunosuppression. We monitored his blood counts, liver and kidney function, and calcium levels closely throughout the treatment.

During the first cycle of chemotherapy, the patient experienced severe neutropenia and required granulocyte colony-stimulating factor (G-CSF) support with Filgrastim to boost his white cell count. He also developed febrile neutropenia, necessitating hospitalization and broad-spectrum antibiotics. Despite these challenges, he completed the first cycle of chemotherapy and antiviral therapy as planned.

Throughout the treatment, we monitored the patient's response with clinical assessments and repeat imaging. After the third cycle of CHOP, a follow-up CT scan showed a partial response with a significant reduction in lymphadenopathy and improvement in his bone lesions. His LDH levels normalized, and hypercalcemia resolved.

However, the patient's clinical course was complicated by persistent infections, and he developed pneumocystis pneumonia (PCP), requiring treatment with Trimethoprim-Sulfamethoxazole and adjunctive corticosteroids. Despite aggressive management, his condition deteriorated due to overwhelming infection and progressive disease.

By the end of the fifth cycle of chemotherapy, the patient's performance status had declined significantly. Repeat imaging and laboratory tests indicated disease progression, with increasing lymphadenopathy, rising LDH levels, and recurrent hypercalcemia. The decision was made to halt further chemotherapy due to his poor tolerance and lack of meaningful response.

Given the progressive nature of his disease and the limited treatment options available, we transitioned the patient to palliative care. His focus shifted to symptom management and improving his quality of life. He was started on oral morphine for pain control, antiemetics for nausea, and continued bisphosphonates to manage hypercalcemia.

The patient's condition continued to decline over the following weeks. Despite maximal supportive care, he developed multi-organ failure and succumbed to his illness approximately eight months after his initial diagnosis.

In retrospect, this case highlights the aggressive nature of ATLL and the challenges in managing this rare and virulent form of T-cell lymphoma. Despite the use of combination chemotherapy and antiviral therapy, the prognosis remains poor, particularly in the acute subtype. Early detection and innovative treatment strategies are essential to improving outcomes in patients with ATLL. This case also underscores the importance of supportive care and the need for a multidisciplinary approach in managing complex oncological diseases.

Continue with
DIAGNOSIS: RARE MEDICAL CASES: VOLUME 3

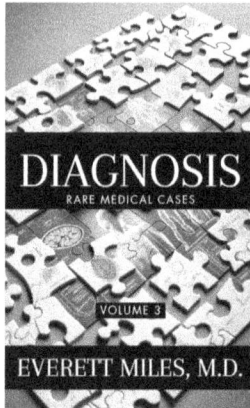

ABOUT THE AUTHOR

Dr. Everett Miles, MD, is a renowned physician with over twenty years of experience in internal medicine and diagnostics. Known for his expertise in solving complex medical cases, Dr. Miles has dedicated his career to unraveling the mysteries of rare diseases. A graduate of Johns Hopkins University School of Medicine, he combines his clinical practice with a passion for medical writing, aiming to educate and inspire both professionals and enthusiasts. Through his series, *Diagnosis: Rare Medical Cases*, Dr. Miles shares his vast knowledge and unique insights, highlighting the art and science of medicine.

www.ingramcontent.com/pod-product-compliance
Lightning Source LLC
Chambersburg PA
CBHW022038190326
41520CB00008B/638